D0191380

Sinusitis Relief

Sinusitis
Relief

HARVEY PLASSE, M.D., and
SHELAGH RYAN MASLINE

AN OWL BOOK
HENRY HOLT AND COMPANY
NEW YORK

The information contained in this book is not intended
as a substitute for consulting with a physician.
All matters regarding your health
require medical supervision.

Henry Holt and Company, LLC
Publishers since 1866
115 West 18th Street
New York, New York 10011

Henry Holt® is a registered trademark of Henry Holt and Company, LLC.

Library of Congress Cataloging-in-Publication Data

Plasse, Harvey.
   Sinusitis relief / Harvey Plasse and Shelagh Ryan Masline.
       p.   cm.
   Includes index.
   ISBN 0-8050-6805-8 (pbk.)
   1. Sinusitis—Popular works.   I. Masline, Shelagh Ryan.   II. Title.
RF425 .P56 2002
616.2'12—dc21   2002068473

Henry Holt books are available for special promotions and premiums.
For details contact: Director, Special Markets.

First Owl Books Edition 2002

Designed by Oksana Kushnir

Printed in the United States of America
10 9 8 7 6 5 4 3 2 1

To my wife, Roberta, and daughter, Stephanie,
for their advice and support
— HARVEY PLASSE, M.D.

To my focused but fun daughter, Caitlin,
the inspiration for all my work, and
to my always loving and always supportive mother, Eileen
— SHELAGH RYAN MASLINE

CONTENTS

Sinusitis Relief

What Is Sinusitis?

If you're reading this book, you probably picked it up because you or someone you know suffers from sinus problems . . . and you're looking for some answers. Sinusitis, which afflicts more than 30 million people in this country, is one of the most common health problems facing Americans today. Perhaps even more surprising, people who have this disease report more pain, depression, and fatigue in their lives than even those who have heart disease or chronic back pain. Yet because sinusitis is so poorly understood, people often suffer in silence, failing to receive proper diagnosis and treatment.

WHAT IS SINUSITIS?

- *Sinusitis* is the term used to describe sinus disease.
- Because sinus and nasal disease are so closely linked, you may also hear your doctor refer to the two jointly as *rhinosinusitis*. The prefix "rhino," from the Greek, means "nose."

SINUSITIS: A PRIMER

The suffix "itis" means inflammation, and sinusitis is an inflammation of the mucous membranes lining one or more of the hollow sinus cavities in the skull. Sinusitis has grown increasingly common over the course of the last decade or so. Although no one knows exactly why, experts speculate that forces such as increased environmental pollution and immune impairment are at work. But whatever the explanation turns out to be, sinus sufferers in this country are making more than 10 million visits to the doctor each year. As a result, physicians write over 13 million antibiotic prescriptions—adding up to a staggering annual tab of more than $3 billion, and literally millions of days lost yearly from work and school. Still more cases of sinusitis go undiagnosed. People mistakenly believe that their symptoms are due to recurrent allergies or colds when, in fact, they have a common condition that responds extremely well to appropriate treatment.

KEY FACTS ABOUT SINUSITIS

- Sinusitis develops in more than 30 million Americans annually.
- Each year an average of four days of work per person is lost because of acute sinusitis.
- Although chronic sinusitis is not as common as acute sinusitis, it is the most common chronic disease in the United States today, affecting 14 percent of the population.
- Most cases of sinusitis are preceded by a cold.
- Sinusitis is on the rise.

AN OVERLOOKED AND MISUNDERSTOOD DISEASE

While in some cases it is just a minor nuisance, often sinusitis can make life miserable. Particularly frustrating is the fact that because the chronic variety usually presents no obvious symptoms—no fever, no rash—little credibility is given to its sufferers. Consequently, people cope with symptoms such as headaches, nasal congestion, a reduced sense of smell, and facial pain for years, sometimes decades, without finding a solution. The fact is, sinusitis is more than just a runny nose or a stuffed-up head. Chronic or recurrent cases carry a significant risk of complications that can be dangerous and, particularly in people with compromised immune systems, even fatal. Though rare, these complications include blindness and infections of the brain. But even when serious complications do not develop, sinusitis can have a severely negative impact on one's overall quality of life. (Read more about sinusitis and quality-of-life issues later in this chapter.)

Overall, sinusitis is shaping up to be one of the most common and yet, simultaneously, one of the most misunderstood diseases of our era. It is misdiagnosed, overdiagnosed, and underdiagnosed, subject alike to both over- and undertreatment. Even when medical attention is sought, not all doctors know how to make the right diagnosis or appropriately treat sinusitis. Some people undergo unnecessary surgical procedures, while others can't seem to obtain the simple prescription that would rid them of painful symptoms. But once you arm yourself with the proper information about sinusitis—the warning signs to watch for, the right people to turn to, the treatment to expect, and more—you can successfully prevent or control the many serious consequences of this disease.

WHAT CAUSES SINUSITIS?

Infection and inflammation that block the sinus openings (ostia) are the direct causes of sinusitis. Given these circumstances, it comes as no surprise that sinus infection most often follows a common cold. But the chances of developing sinus problems are greatly enhanced by a whole host of other factors, including allergies, immune system problems, polyps, and swollen adenoids. An overall rise in immune impairment is a major contributing factor to the epidemic of sinusitis in recent years, as is the increase in urban air pollution. It is now generally accepted that diseases that are related to or increase the risk for sinusitis are on the rise worldwide and are associated with increased pollution. Another aspect that scientists are focusing on is the role of fungi, which appear to be nearly ubiquitous in the sinuses. Your chances of developing sinus disease may also be greater if you are a smoker, or even if you are exposed to secondhand smoke. Changes in ambient pressure—as during air travel or scuba diving—also contribute to the problem. Some of these factors can be avoided while others are inevitable, for the anatomy of the nasal passages and sinuses themselves plays an occasional role in sinusitis. To further complicate matters, explanations for sinus infection and pain can usually be attributed to a combination of some or all of these elements. (Read more about the causes of sinusitis in chapters 3 and 4.)

THE ANATOMY OF A SINUS INFECTION

Not everyone who has a cold or an allergic reaction develops sinusitis. You are most likely to develop sinusitis when the following three factors are all present:

- You have sinus blockage. This can be the result of inflammation, or of mechanical obstruction such as enlarged adenoids or nasal polyps.
- You are experiencing some kind of immune system impairment.
- Infection-causing microorganisms are present.

Ostial Obstruction

When you experience an inflammatory problem such as an upper respiratory infection or allergic reaction, the diameter of a sinus opening shrinks. Doctors refer to this condition as ostial obstruction. The osteomeatal unit, or OMU, is considered the seat of sinus disease, since the majority of the sinuses drain into this area around the nose. Sinusitis is usually initiated with obstruction of this final common pathway.

The Inflammatory Response

Inflammation is most commonly due to viral infection or allergies. The resulting redness, swelling, heat, and pain are local tissue reactions to an abnormal stimulus (such as infection, allergy, injury, or irritation). The inflammatory response is actually a protective move on the part of your body to isolate the affected area and rush in blood packed with disease-fighting antibodies to neutralize any hostile invaders. Yet inflammation leads to acute rhinitis: a sudden swelling of the mucous membrane that lines the nose. As the swelling extends to the sinus membranes, it increasingly interferes with airflow and normal mucous drainage, eventually narrowing the ostia or even closing them altogether.

The Role of Colds and Allergies

Colds and allergies are the most common culprits responsible for inflammation and obstructed drainage. If these are ruled out, your physician will examine your nose and sinuses for signs of anatomic or mechanical obstruction. For example, small grapelike growths called nasal polyps can interfere with the normal drainage of your sinuses. Other possible causes of obstruction include unusually small drainage openings, a significantly deviated septum, and tumors. Adequate mucociliary clearance—the sweeping of mucus through sinus chambers by microscopic hairs called cilia—is also essential to proper drainage and the normal functioning of the sinuses. Finally, a change in the nature or amount of secretions within the nasal cavities may lead to inadequate drainage. Sinusitis develops when inflammation is strong enough to impair local immune defenses as well as contribute to ostial obstruction.

Immune Impairment

The immune system is the body's natural defense against infection. In the nose and sinuses—indeed, throughout the respiratory system—mucous secretions are rich in substances that destroy or inhibit disease-causing microorganisms. Among the most important of these are proteins known as immunoglobulins. These vital antibodies work to eradicate infectious organisms that play a significant role in sinusitis. Other protective substances in mucus are T cells, which are best known for their ability to combat HIV infection. In addition, there are enzymes that attack *Candida* and other fungi and kill bacteria by invading and digesting their walls. Current research supports a greater emphasis on the role of weakened immune defenses in chronic sinusitis, shifting away somewhat from the traditional focus on infection. It may be that the presence of disease-causing organisms is less significant than the weakened immune system that makes a person susceptible to them.

A Greater Susceptibility to Disease

When your immune system is functioning at peak efficiency, disease-fighting substances band together to help keep you healthy. But if your body no longer produces an adequate number of antibodies, you become more susceptible to a whole panoply of disorders—and featuring prominently among these is sinusitis. Immune impairment can have any number of different causes. For example, if you are undergoing aggressive chemotherapy for cancer or are taking cortisone for a chronic condition such as colitis, your immune system is weakened. This makes you more likely to come down with a cold or flu that can be a precursor to sinusitis. Sinus disease is also especially common in people with weakened immune systems due to HIV infection. In recent years, the overuse of broad-spectrum antibiotics has contributed to impaired immunity by encouraging the emergence of drug-resistant strains of bacteria. Along with the increases in air pollution and the corresponding increase in allergic rhinitis, this practice is believed to be a major contributing factor to the soaring incidence of sinusitis.

The Overuse of Antibiotics

Over the course of the last decade or two, there has been an explosion of so-called supergerms or superbugs, bacteria that cause infections that are difficult and sometimes impossible to treat with the antibiotics we have available today. Supergerms are a direct consequence of the overuse of antibiotics. To set the record straight, antibiotics are only effective in curing bacterial infections; they have no effect whatsoever on viruses. Nevertheless, patients frequently ask for and doctors often continue to prescribe these drugs for viral infections such as colds and flu. Incredibly, the Centers for Disease Control and Prevention (CDC) estimate that one-third of the 150 million outpatient prescriptions written for antibiotics in the United States each year is unnecessary. To further complicate matters, livestock on farms are routinely fed antibiotics to prevent infection and promote growth. Scientists are concerned that this practice will eventually lead to drug-resistant bacteria that can reach us through the food chain.

Inside your body, bacteria adapt to the onslaught of repeated antibiotic attacks by morphing into ever newer, tougher, and harder-to-treat strains. Antibiotics may also destroy the friendly bacteria that normally reside in your digestive tract, thus opening the door to the growth of the more destructive *Candida* fungus. The irony is that treatment with the same antibiotics that miraculously cure many dangerous bacterial infections can also lead to the generation of virulent supergerms. Indeed, these are often the very bacteria responsible for serious and persistent cases of chronic sinusitis that fail to respond to regular antibiotic treatment. The answer? According to organizations such as the CDC and the American Medical Association (AMA), it lies in reducing the number of unnecessary antibiotic prescriptions and educating the public about the differences between viral and bacterial infections. As an individual, you can protect yourself and your family by talking to your own physician and making certain that he or she prescribes antibiotics only when absolutely necessary. Even though they are more expensive, you might also consider buying free-range, antibiotic-free chicken and beef.

Bacteria and Other Disease-Causing Microorganisms

The third critical element in the initiation of sinusitis is the presence of bacteria or other disease-causing microorganisms. Sinusitis is an infection, frequently brought on by a virus such as a cold or flu, but usually perpetuated by bacteria, and occasionally by a fungus. Bacteria are opportunistic invaders that take advantage of other weakened conditions of the body—in this case, sinus obstruction and immune impairment. Most often, inflammation due to viral infection or allergy is a key component in this process; blocking the ostia, it leads to poor sinus drainage. But whether blockage is due to inflammation or mechanical problems (such as polyps or adenoids), once the sinuses can no longer drain properly, pus, mucus, and other secretions begin to accumulate in cavities. This creates a fertile breeding ground for infectious microorganisms such as bacteria and fungi. The vicious cycle of sinusitis is thus begun, as inflammation that blocks airflow and drainage opens the door to infection, which in turn causes further inflammation and blockage, and so on until the cycle is finally broken by the body's own immune defenses or through medical intervention.

BACTERIAL CAUSES OF SINUSITIS

A major difference between acute and chronic sinus disease lies in the types of organisms involved. Three out of four cases of acute disease are caused by *Streptococcus pneumoniae* or *Hemophilus influenzae* bacteria. Anaerobes—stubborn bacteria that live and grow in the absence of oxygen—are commonly found in chronic sinusitis, although it is uncertain whether this is a cause or effect of the disease. Multiple organisms are also more likely to be involved in chronic infections.

THE DIFFERENT TYPES OF SINUSITIS

To clarify some of the confusion and misperceptions that persist concerning sinusitis, doctors make careful distinctions among the different types of this disease. Specifically, they categorize sinusitis according to which cavities are affected and how long symptoms last. There are four pairs of sinuses: the maxillary, frontal, ethmoid, and sphenoid. (Read more about the anatomy of the sinuses in chapter 2.) The location of sinus pain and swelling depends upon which sinuses are affected. For example, if you have a maxillary infection, your teeth and upper jaw may ache. In contrast, an infection of the frontal sinuses in the forehead causes pain when this area is touched.

Perhaps even more important, physicians make a careful distinction between two major categories of sinusitis: acute and chronic. Both forms of sinusitis can be confusing to diagnose and treat. *Acute sinusitis* most commonly occurs as a complication of a common cold, but may also be linked with allergies, anatomic abnormalities, or even dental infection. Because they are similar and often overlap, acute sinusitis is often confused with a cold, and thus can be neglected by affected individuals or incorrectly treated by doctors. When this happens, the result can be chronic sinusitis, the symptoms of which are far more subtle and even trickier to diagnose.

By definition, acute sinusitis lasts up to four weeks. Within that time, there is a complete resolution of symptoms such as congestion, postnasal drip, and headache. However, if symptoms linger longer than this, you may have or be at risk of developing *chronic sinusitis*. In the long run, chronic disease exacts a much deadlier toll on the sinuses. Chronic sinusitis occurs when symptoms persist for twelve weeks or longer. People who suffer from chronic sinusitis may never feel completely right. They always have what seems like a slight cold or nasal congestion, which occasionally flares up into full-blown sinus infection.

There are also two further subdivisions of sinusitis. *Subacute sinusitis* occurs when symptoms last longer than four but less than twelve weeks. It is especially important to correctly diagnose and treat this type of problem, before it becomes chronic and causes permanent scarring and narrowing of the sinuses. *Recurrent acute sinusitis* consists of four or more acute episodes in one year. Between these attacks, there are no symptoms. Although sinusitis—no matter what type—is most commonly due to bacterial infection, it may also be caused by a fungus or virus. In the case of recurrent sinusitis, you may be infected by different microorganisms at different times.

ACUTE SINUSITIS

Most cases of sinus disease are acute sinusitis. That is, they either respond to treatment or clear up on their own within four weeks. Say

---

THE FOUR TYPES OF SINUSITIS

- Acute sinusitis lasts up to four weeks, during which time there is a complete resolution of symptoms.
- Subacute sinusitis lasts longer than four weeks, but less than twelve weeks.
- Recurrent acute sinusitis consists of four or more acute episodes within one year.
- Chronic sinusitis lasts twelve weeks or longer.

---

you've developed a cold that lasts longer than usual. You have trouble breathing through your nose, and at night a persistent cough disturbs your sleep. To make matters even worse, your sinuses are achy and tender to the touch. In fact, the problem may not be a cold at all—you probably have acute sinusitis.

Sinusitis and the Common Cold

Acute sinusitis is most commonly preceded by a common cold, which physicians refer to as viral rhinitis. Only a small percentage of people with colds go on to develop acute sinusitis. However, because cold and flu viruses are so prevalent, especially in the winter months, millions of Americans develop sinusitis each year.

Normal mucous production, intact mucous membranes, good mucociliary clearance, and open ostia are all essential to proper sinus drainage. But nearly nine out of ten people experience sinus cavity abnormalities when they have a cold. As we mentioned earlier, the most common problem is blockage of the osteomeatal unit (OMU), the area around the nose into which the majority of the sinuses drain. Blockage of the OMU accompanies almost all upper respiratory infections and sets off the chain of events that initiates sinusitis. When this inflammatory pathway is activated, a number of different things take place. Blood vessels in the nasal turbinates become swollen and engorged; plasma leaks into the nose and sinuses; mucociliary clearance becomes impaired; mucosal gas metabolism changes; goblet cells and seromucous glands produce excess mucus; secretions thicken and stagnate; and pain nerves and/or sneeze and cough reflexes are stimulated. In other words, ostial blockage and other factors lead to infection in one or more cavities, and you develop acute sinusitis. (Read about the role of upper respiratory infections in greater detail in chapter 3.)

REQUIREMENTS FOR NORMAL SINUS DRAINAGE
- Normal mucous production
- Intact mucous membranes
- Proper mucociliary clearance
- Open, unblocked ostia

The Signs and Symptoms of Acute Sinusitis

If you have a cold that persists for ten days or longer, chances are you have an acute sinus infection. Common symptoms include congestion, nasal discharge, postnasal drip, and a reduced or absent sense of smell (hyposmia or anosmia). Nasal discharge may remain clear, or become yellow or green. Sometimes the discharge is tinged with blood due to the drying out of delicate mucous membranes or overzealous nose blowing. Postnasal drip may cause hoarseness, a sore throat, and cough. Because mucus trickles down your windpipe and bronchial tubes while you sleep, your cough will probably be worse at night and early in the morning. In some cases, postnasal drip is so severe that it causes gagging and vomiting in the morning. Many people also suffer from low-grade fever, chills, night sweats, and fatigue. Bad breath (halitosis) is a minor but inconvenient problem for some. Of course, complicating diagnosis is the fact that many of these same signs and symptoms also occur in colds.

Headache and Facial Pain

Most people with acute sinus disease suffer from headache or facial pain. In fact, these hallmark symptoms often help physicians distinguish cases of sinusitis from simple colds and flu, especially when pain regularly occurs at certain times of the day. Sinus headaches cause deep, dull pain that ranges from mild to moderate intensity. Pain may be due to inflammation, or pressure within the sinuses brought on by trapped air, or an accumulation of undrained fluid. Air may also be blocked from entering a sinus, creating a vacuum. People with vacuum-type sinus headaches are sensitive to pressure changes such as those that occur in low-pressure weather systems or when descending in an airplane. They may also experience sensations of ear pain, pressure, or fullness.

The Location of Sinus Pain

The location of pain depends on which sinuses are infected. When the frontals are involved, pain is in the forehead and over the eyes. Maxillary pain frequently occurs between the cheek and nose, but may also affect the upper teeth. Many people who have a maxillary infection believe toothache is the problem, and they initially consult a dentist rather than a doctor. Maxillary pain may also be referred to the ear or back of the head. Ethmoid infection often accompanies maxillary as well as other types of sinusitis. Infected ethmoid sinuses produce pain between and behind the eyes. Since the ethmoids are located near the tear ducts in the corners of the eyes, there may also be swelling of the eyelids and surrounding tissues. The eyes themselves may ache and water. Sphenoid sinuses, which are located deep within the skull, can cause pain just about anywhere on the head. (Note: The symptoms of sinusitis often differ for children. For instance, headaches are uncommon in youngsters—especially those under age six. Turn to chapter 8 to read about sinusitis in children.)

WHERE DOES IT HURT?

- Acute frontal sinusitis causes a severe frontal headache and tenderness of the involved sinus in the forehead.
- Acute maxillary sinusitis causes pain, pressure, and tenderness over the cheekbone. There may also be toothache and temporal headache.
- Acute ethmoid sinusitis causes a persistent headache around the eyes or in the forehead.
- Acute sphenoid sinusitis causes diffuse headache pain around the skull and is often accompanied by a fever.

Diagnosing Acute Sinusitis

Physicians make a diagnosis of acute sinusitis when you have:

- Two or more major factors
- One major and two minor factors
- Nasal purulence on examination

A diagnosis of acute sinusitis is suggested when you have:

- One major sign or symptom
- Two or more minor signs or symptoms

Major Factors:
- Facial pain or pressure
- Facial congestion or fullness
- Nasal obstruction and congestion
- Nasal discharge, which can be purulent, discolored postnasal drainage
- Reduced or absent sense of smell (hyposmia or anosmia)
- Fever
- Purulence in nasal cavity on examination

Minor Factors:
- Headache
- Fatigue
- Bad breath (halitosis)
- Dental pain
- Cough
- Ear pain, pressure, or fullness

SUBACUTE AND RECURRENT ACUTE SINUSITIS

Keep in mind that there are also two important subcategories of acute sinusitis: subacute and recurrent acute. If symptoms persist for longer than four but less than twelve weeks, you have what is known as subacute sinusitis. Again, it is essential to stop subacute disease dead in its tracks—otherwise, it can progress to the chronic stage, which is associated with permanent scarring and narrowing of the sinuses.

Subacute follows acute sinusitis, and its symptoms are more subtle. You may no longer be in severe discomfort, but neither are you back to your normal, healthy self. Symptoms generally include intermittent nasal congestion and a cloudy discharge, which may (unlike the acute variety) affect only one side of the nose or head. Many people also experience a mild headache or sore throat, especially in the morning, as a result of nighttime postnasal drip. If you find yourself with symptoms like these following an acute episode of sinusitis, see your doctor. Vigorous treatment with antibiotics can prevent more serious future damage.

When you experience four or more acute attacks within one year (without any symptoms in between), you have recurrent acute sinusitis. Some people are more prone to periodic sinus attacks than others. For example, if you have a form of immune impairment (such as HIV) or sinus dysfunction (such as narrowed sinus openings due to scarring), you may often develop an acute flare-up following a cold or flu. Of course, no two cases of sinusitis are exactly alike, and the causes of acute attacks vary from person to person. Potential triggers include anxiety, depression, stress, sleep disturbances, hormonal changes associated with pregnancy or PMS, drinking too much alcohol, smoking cigarettes, and breathing in irritating secondhand smoke, dust, or paint. Susceptible individuals may also develop sinusitis from changes in ambient pressure, as when flying or scuba diving. Variations in temperature and weather can also play a role, as when you get chilled or overheated, are caught in the rain, or sleep in a draft. Molds or fungi that flourish in damp basements are yet another cause. Flare-ups of recurrent acute sinusitis generally last only a week or two, but may require antibiotic treatment.

CHRONIC SINUSITIS

In recent years, there has been a significant change in the understanding of chronic sinus disease. Whereas not too long ago it was seen primarily as an infectious problem, today researchers are focusing more attention on the immunological aspects. Although far less prevalent than acute disease, chronic sinusitis is the most common chronic illness in the United States today. Moreover, due to factors such as the increase in air pollutants and the corresponding rise in allergic rhinitis, the overuse of antibiotics, and the overall increase in immune impairment, the incidence of chronic sinusitis is rapidly increasing to epidemic proportions. Of particular concern are serious complications—especially those that affect the eyes and brain—that are most frequently associated with chronic disease.

The Signs and Symptoms of Chronic Sinusitis

In chronic sinusitis, signs and symptoms by definition last for twelve weeks or longer. They commonly include chronic mild to moderate discomfort, nasal congestion, postnasal drip, a decrease or loss of the sense of smell, and a low-grade fever. Some people also experience a

WHY IS ALLERGIC RHINITIS ON THE RISE?

There are several theories about the recent rise in allergic rhinitis:

- Many experts believe that it is due to the increase in diesel fuel in the air. They point out that both allergic rhinitis and asthma are more common in the industrialized societies of the United States and Europe. These problems are relatively rare in the non-Western world, especially among children.
- Another theory associates the increase in allergic rhinitis—along with atopic allergy and asthma—with the decrease in childhood infections. Over the years, vaccinations, smaller family size, and antibiotics have combined to reduce the frequency of common childhood diseases ranging from mumps and measles to colds and flu. But infections are thought to stimulate a nonatopic type of immune system. In their absence, children develop immune systems that are more prone to allergic rhinitis and asthma.

sore throat, cough, bad breath, or extreme fatigue. But even though these signs and symptoms are roughly the same as those describing acute sinusitis, in the chronic variety they are less dramatic and more subtle. This poses a unique set of problems for chronic sinusitis sufferers. Even though you may feel sluggish and ill, your spouse or employer or teacher may not take your disease seriously. Indeed, some regular medical practitioners find it challenging to recognize the understated signs and symptoms of chronic sinusitis. Nevertheless, it is essential to accurately diagnose and treat sinus disease that lasts for a prolonged period of time—otherwise, it can cause permanent damage and destruction of sinus tissues. In diagnosis, doctors must carefully distinguish chronic sinusitis from other ailments with similar signs and symptoms, such as colds, allergies, and bronchitis. (Turn to chapter 3 to learn more about the links among sinusitis, respiratory infections, allergies, and asthma.)

Diagnosing Chronic Sinusitis

The signs and symptoms of chronic sinusitis are more or less the same as those of the acute illness. However, they are more subtle and tend to drag on and on. A diagnosis of chronic sinusitis is made when you have two or more major factors, or one major and two minor factors, or purulence on nasal examination.

Major Factors:
- Facial pain or pressure
- Nasal obstruction and congestion
- Nasal discharge and purulence, discolored postnasal discharge
- Facial congestion or fullness
- Reduced or absent sense of smell (hyposmia or anosmia)
- Purulence in nasal cavity on examination

Minor Factors:
- Headache
- Fever
- Fatigue
- Dental pain
- Ear pain, pressure, or fullness
- Bad breath (halitosis)
- Cough

THE COMPLICATIONS OF SINUSITIS

Although physicians have made great strides in controlling sinus disease, serious complications still can and do occur. Of course, hands down, acute sinusitis that progresses to chronic disease is the most common complication and one that you must make every effort to avoid. It is also possible for painful, fluid-filled cysts to develop and become infected. In some cases, a maxillary sinus infection extends to the upper teeth. Rare complications include the spread of infection into the pituitary gland or even into the blood (bacteremia). The sinus complications that are of greatest concern to physicians are those that occur when infection extends beyond the bony walls of the sinuses into the nearby vital structures of the eyes and brain. (Turn to chapter 7 to learn more about eye and brain complications.) But even if you don't develop serious complications, sinusitis can have a dramatic negative impact on your quality of life.

SINUSITIS AND QUALITY OF LIFE

Whenever you suffer from sinusitis—or related colds or allergies—symptoms such as a runny nose, congestion, cough, and fatigue can make you feel downright miserable. But what many people fail to realize is that these conditions can also impair your overall quality of life. Sinusitis impacts not only the physical but also the emotional functioning of affected individuals. Over time, physical discomforts may come to have an effect on your relationships at home and work. If you feel lousy and can't sleep at night, you may find yourself being irritable and impatient with family members. Things that you used to let go may now make you lash out in anger. At work, you may not be able to think as clearly as usual or be as productive. And if you break into a sneezing fit, or can't keep your eyes open during an important meeting, the embarrassment can be considerable. If this happens on a consistent basis and is accompanied by multiple absences—as is often the case with chronic sinusitis—you may be at risk of losing your job. Affected children frequently miss school, leading to academic and social difficulties. Even when they attend classes, discomfort and exhaustion may make it hard to concentrate on math or reading—and a child suffering from chronic sinusitis may not be up to participating in gym class at all. Further complicating matters is the fact that medications you take to control symptoms can actually add to the problem, alternately causing side effects such as drowsiness and lethargy or nervousness and insomnia. Over time, these sorts of experiences can lead to a diminished self-image and depression.

The Impact of Chronic Sinusitis

Of the various sinus and nasal problems, long-lasting chronic sinusitis has the greatest negative impact on physical and emotional functioning. Indeed, studies have shown that its effects are comparable to those of other serious health problems, including congestive heart failure and recent heart attacks. Most people with chronic sinusitis always feel a little under the weather—they are worn out and tired and usually congested. A few experience nearly constant headaches and sinus pain. Yet because these symptoms are more subtle and less dramatic than those of a bad cold or acute sinusitis or an allergy attack, family members, employers, and teachers are not always sympathetic and understanding—which can be extremely frustrating.

People with chronic sinusitis also get sick more often than other people. When you already have a weakened immune system from fighting off disease, you are more susceptible to coming down with a cold or succumbing to an allergic reaction. Even worse, a minor cold or allergic reaction is more likely to explode into a case of full-blown sinusitis. Consequently, chronic sinusitis sufferers miss more days of work or school and are usually compelled to make frequent visits to the doctor.

Chronic sinusitis is also more apt to cause disturbing alterations in the senses of smell and taste. Changes in smell may include a decreased (or even absent) sense of smell and the sensation of phantom odors. As a result, some people feel anxiety about safety issues, such as detecting fire or gas leaks, or eating spoiled food; others express self-conscious concern about their breath and body odor. Changes in smell are often accompanied by changes in taste—such as an altered taste for food, less enjoyment from eating, and a sudden preference for spicier foods. Not surprisingly, all these effects often add up to a reduced enjoyment of life. In studies, chronic sinusitis sufferers typically report less satisfaction with their lives than healthy individuals.

HOW COLDS, ALLERGIES, AND SINUSITIS MAY AFFECT YOUR LIFE

- Sleep disturbances
- Diminished sense of smell and taste
- Cognitive impairment
- Lost productivity
- Absences from work or school
- Inability to fully participate in sports and other physical activities
- Diminished self-image

UNDERSTANDING SINUSITIS

Clearly, sinusitis can have a major impact on every aspect of your life. As a result, it is essential to understand more about this troubling disease, so you know what to do if you or a loved one experiences its symptoms. Now that you've learned the basics about the disease itself, in the next chapter we'll take a closer look at the anatomy of the sinuses.

CHAPTER 2

All About the Sinuses

In order to fully understand sinusitis, it is important to step back for a moment and learn more about the sinuses themselves: what they are, where they are located, and how they function in the human body. (Interestingly, this last question is something of a mystery even to doctors and researchers!) The sinuses are air-filled cavities in the skull bones situated around the nose and eyes. Physicians commonly refer to them as paranasal sinuses. When people complain that they are having a sinus attack, they usually mean that they are experiencing symptoms in one or more sinus cavities. Since the sinuses are close to many other vital structures in the body, it is essential to control sinusitis before serious complications develop.

VITAL STRUCTURES NEAR THE SINUSES

- Brain
- Orbits (eye sockets)
- Optic nerves (nerves that transmit information about visual images from the retina of the eye to the brain)
- Tear ducts
- Teeth
- Carotid arteries (the two principal arteries that carry blood from the aorta to the head)

The Four Pairs of Sinuses

There are four pairs of sinuses, named after the bones in which they are found: the frontal, maxillary, ethmoid, and sphenoid. The pairs are roughly divided in half for each side of the head, although the halves are not necessarily symmetrical. That is, they may vary in size and shape. Occasionally, one or sometimes even both sinuses are missing from a pair. Although this is relatively uncommon, it happens most frequently with the frontal sinuses. The ethmoids differ from the other sinuses in that they consist of a number of very small cavities.

THE FOUR SINUSES

- Frontal sinuses over the eyes in the brow area
- Maxillary sinuses inside the cheekbones
- Ethmoid sinuses just behind the bridge of the nose and between the eyes
- Sphenoid sinuses behind the ethmoids in the upper region of the nose and behind the eyes

---

A Part of the Respiratory System

Like the mouth, nose, throat, airways, and lungs, the sinuses are part of the body's respiratory system. The respiratory system is responsible for the exchange of oxygen and carbon dioxide of the air, blood, and body tissues. The circulatory system, consisting of the heart and blood vessels, makes certain that oxygen reaches cells and that the waste product carbon dioxide is carried away. Oxygen is used by cells throughout the body to produce energy.

The Sinuses and the Nose: A Close Connection

When a person is healthy, mucus and air pass continuously through narrow channels, or ducts, that lead from the sinuses to the back of the nose. At the end of each channel, air and mucus travel through tiny holes or openings known as ostia. The channels are lined with a mucous membrane called respiratory epithelium. This is swept clean on a continuous basis by tiny beating hairs called cilia, in a process known as mucociliary clearance. The ciliary beat also transports the mucous blanket (composed of mucus and to a lesser degree other fluids) through the sinuses.

Although the sinuses themselves are normally free from bacteria, their close connection with the nose means that the impact of any

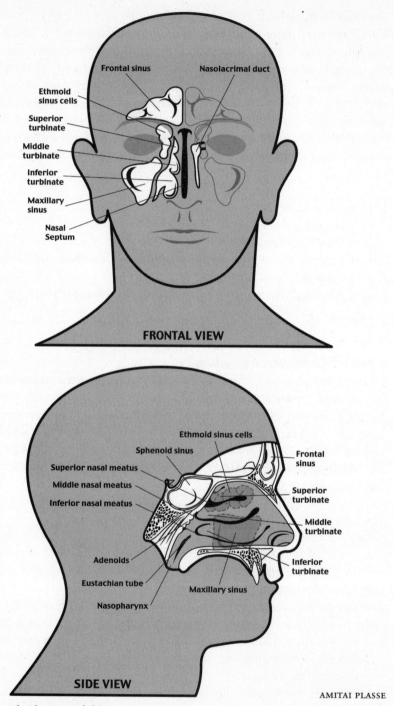

Front and side view of the sinuses.

problem that causes swelling in the nasal cavity—such as an upper respiratory infection (cold or flu) or allergic reaction—can partially or completely block the ostia, causing sinus problems. In fact, while in this book we consistently use the term *sinusitis,* physicians often jointly refer to sinus and nasal problems as rhinosinusitis. This is because the two are so closely linked that it is sometimes difficult to distinguish between them.

NORMAL DRAINAGE: AN ESSENTIAL ELEMENT OF SINUS HEALTH

In healthy people, as much as a quart of mucus passes through the four sets of sinuses each day. Mucus is drained through the tiny ostia, several of which are located—somewhat illogically from a plumbing perspective—at the top of sinuses. When an ostium is blocked by inflammation, an excess of undrained mucus leads to stuffiness, discomfort, and in some cases infection.

The warm and moist hollow air spaces of the sinuses provide particularly fertile breeding grounds for infectious organisms. When the cilia fail to continuously sweep the sinuses clear, undrained mucus can accumulate and become infected with bacteria or other microorganisms. Thriving bacteria lead to problems such as infection within the closed spaces. The nature and location of sinus pain and swelling varies according to which sinuses are infected.

WHAT HEALTHY SINUSES NEED

In order to remain healthy and disease-free, the sinuses require three factors:

- Normal, intact physical structures, including patent (unobstructed) ostia
- Normal mucociliary clearance
- Normal quantity and quality of secretions

THE MAXILLARY SINUSES

Located inside each cheekbone between the eyes and upper teeth, these two pyramid-shaped cavities are the largest sinuses. Small maxillary sinuses are present at birth. They enlarge rapidly until age three, and again between ages seven and twelve, until they are fully developed in adulthood. The maxillary sinuses play a large part in childhood sinusitis as well as adult sinusitis. Often they are slightly larger in males.

The maxillary sinuses arise from and drain into small channels called the middle meati, which are located on either side of the nose under the shelter of a bone called the middle turbinate (one of three mucous-membrane-covered bones that arise from the nasal walls). The maxillaries drain through ostia at the top of the sinus, a location that can lead to drainage problems. In some cases, there are also secondary openings due to infection or surgery. For example, a maxillary sinus infection occasionally ruptures a very thin membrane called the fontanelle, creating another permanent sinus opening. When a primary ostium becomes blocked, a secondary opening can be helpful in the transfer of mucus and air. However, the benefits are limited, because the cilia are programmed to sweep mucus toward the primary drainage opening.

How the Maxillary Sinuses Drain

Maxillary sinus flow has a unique pattern. The mucous blanket travels along a well-defined pathway that is probably genetically predetermined. The cilia in maxillary cavities propel the mucus in a starlike pattern around the circumference of the sinus, to the ostium, through the infundibulum into the middle meatus, and finally into the nasal cavity.

THE FRONTAL SINUSES

These second-largest sinuses lie over the eyes in the brow area, in what is called the frontal bone. The frontals are very tiny at birth, fairly developed by age twelve, and reach their full size before the age of twenty. In some cases, one of the frontal sinuses may be congenitally underdeveloped or missing altogether. This occurs more often than you might think—in fact, in more than one in ten people.

The frontal sinuses arise from and drain into small channels called the middle meati, which are located on either side of the nose beneath the middle turbinate. Because frontal anatomy varies, some people are more apt to develop problems with these sinuses than others. For example, the mucous blanket may encounter swelling, small mucosal defects, or bony crests within the frontal sinus. Sometimes it is able to

WHAT ARE THE TURBINATES?

- The turbinates are spiral-shaped, spongy bones on the outer walls of the nasal passages on either side of the nose. Because of their shell-like shape, they are also known as concha.
- There are generally three turbinates: the inferior (lower), middle, and superior (upper). In some cases, a small supreme turbinate is also present.
- The turbinates are lined with respiratory epithelium, which is rich in mucous-secreting goblet cells.
- As you inhale, the turbinates warm, humidify, and filter the air you take in. They also protect the sinus drainage and tear duct openings.
- The turbinates are rich in antibodies and react to inhaled allergens and irritants with an acute or chronic increase in tissue size. This is known as a hypertrophic change.
- The nasal lining swells and shrinks in a cyclical pattern several times each day. This is called the nasal cycle. The normal intermittent congestion of this cycle is sometimes mistaken for the permanent thickening seen in chronic sinusitis.
- Airflow varies as a result of turbinate size.

bypass these obstacles. On other occasions, secretions are temporarily retained until the mucous blanket is able to move onward.

How the Frontal Sinuses Drain

The frontal sinuses are unique in that they are the only sinuses in which mucus travels around the sinus in a circular pattern, encompassing both sides, the roof, and the floor of the cavity. Mucus and debris may therefore recycle through the frontal sinus many times, before at last exiting into the middle meatus and out to the nasal cavity.

THE SPHENOID SINUSES

The sphenoids, which are the third-largest sinuses, are located in the upper region of the nose. These sinuses are not present at birth, but first develop at age three and are extensively developed by age seven. Since the sphenoids lie deep within the skull, they have traditionally been difficult to examine. In consequence, prior to modern methods of evaluation and treatment, infections in these chambers were apt to go undiagnosed until they caused serious problems. Hence the sphenoids earned their nickname "the neglected sinuses." Today, using a variety of state-of-the-art imaging techniques such as CT scanning, doctors can more readily detect and treat sphenoid infections.

How the Sphenoid Sinuses Drain

The drainage openings of the sphenoids are near those of the posterior ethmoids. Like the maxillary sinus, the sphenoid sinus depends on mucociliary flow for drainage, since the ostium is typically located 10 to 15 millimeters above the floor of the sinus.

THE ETHMOID SINUSES

The ethmoids lie behind the maxillaries and between the bony orbits of the eyes. These complex labyrinths of tiny air pockets are present at birth and almost fully mature by the age of twelve. In adults, the ethmoid sinuses form a pyramid. Between seven and fifteen cavities on each side of the head drain into tiny openings in the nose. The ethmoids are divided into two categories: anterior and posterior. The posterior chambers are usually larger and fewer in number.

The ethmoids are separated from the eye sockets or orbits by only paper-thin walls known as lamina papyracea. Because of this close proximity, ethmoid sinuses are most likely to be associated with eye-related complications, ranging from simple infections to blindness. Ethmoid surgery also carries a greater risk of eye injuries than other types of sinus procedures, since there is sometimes only a thin layer of bone or even a lack of bone dividing their cavities from the orbit or optic nerve. When ethmoid sinuses extend beneath the eye, they can cause blockage and infection of the maxillary sinus. If they expand into the middle turbinate bone in the nose, the turbinate may become a cause of infection.

How the Ethmoid Sinuses Drain

- The anterior ethmoid sinuses drain into the middle meati, small channels on either side of the nose tucked under the middle turbinate. From there they proceed into the nasal cavity.
- The posterior ethmoid sinuses drain into the superior and supreme meati. From there they proceed into a small pocket called the sphenoethmoidal recess, and onward into the naso-

pharynx (the passage connecting the cavity behind the nose to the top of the throat).

THE OSTEOMEATAL UNIT

The maxillary, frontal, and anterior ethmoid sinuses all arise from and drain into a small channel called the middle meatus. The middle meatus and adjacent middle meatal structures are known as the osteomeatal unit, or OMU. (This is also referred to as the osteomeatal complex, or OMC.) The OMU is not a discrete anatomic structure. Instead, it is a functional term used by physicians to discuss the disease process of sinusitis.

The OMU collectively includes the following structures: the uncinate process; the ethmoid infundibulum; anterior ethmoid cells; and the ostia of the anterior ethmoid, maxillary, and frontal sinuses. Obstruction in this critical region can lead to frontal, maxillary, or anterior ethmoid sinusitis. Since the anterior ethmoids, frontal sinuses, and maxillary sinuses all drain into the OMU, this area is considered to be the seat of sinus disease. In order to cure an OMU-related problem, a doctor may be required to treat all three sinuses.

ABOUT THE OSTEOMEATAL UNIT

- The osteomeatal unit (OMU) is the name for the area into which the anterior ethmoid, maxillary, and frontal sinuses all drain.
- Obstruction in this critical region can lead to anterior ethmoid, maxillary, or frontal sinusitis.
- As a result, this area is considered to be the seat of sinus disease. It is also referred to as the final common pathway in the development of sinusitis.

THE RESPIRATORY EPITHELIUM

The sinuses, nose, and lungs all have the same type of lining, or respiratory epithelium, that serves as an active barrier to infectious bacteria and other microorganisms. The thickness of the sinus lining as a whole varies from 0.2 to 0.8 millimeter, although it is uniform within each cavity. The goblet cells and mucoserous glands that line the sinuses—along with those in the nose—secrete a pint or more a day of clear, clean mucus. This produces a protective mucous blanket.

The Mucous Blanket

The mucous blanket provides important local immunologic defense. A breakdown in this defense is one of three factors (along with ostial obstruction and the presence of disease-causing bacteria) that can lead to sinusitis. In normal, healthy sinuses, the mucous blanket is composed of two layers, the inner one of which is lined with thousands of tiny projecting hairs called cilia.

MUCOCILIARY CLEARANCE

The constant sweeping action of cilia helps keep the sinuses free from bacteria and other microorganisms. This facilitates the normal production and flow of mucus around the nasal passages—that is, mucociliary clearance. Tiny respiratory cilia are responsible for transporting mucus, as well as for trapping inhaled particles and bacteria. Even though the effective action of the cilia helps keep the sinuses free from infectious microorganisms, the cilia do not actually keep the sinuses sterile. Researchers today believe that there are always some fungi residing in even normal sinuses. (In contrast, overgrowth of fungi or excessive reaction to fungi is due to disease. Read more about fungus infection and sinusitis in chapter 4.)

When Mucociliary Clearance Is Impaired

When the cilia cannot function properly, sinus drainage is impaired. Factors contributing to this problem may include inadequate oxygen availability (hypoxia), changes in temperature, dehydration, medications such as antihistamines, environmental irritants, cigarette smoke, and foreign bodies. Trauma, tumors, allergens, infection, and diseases such as cystic fibrosis may also affect sinus drainage. In an acute case of sinusitis with a great deal of mucous secretion, ciliary activity is often damaged or even absent—yet the cilia resume their normal tasks when the infection is cured. On the other hand, if you suffer from chronic sinusitis over a long period of time, your cilia may suffer longer-lasting (even permanent) damage, resulting in an inability to clear secretions from the sinuses.

WHY DO WE HAVE SINUSES?

Over the years, many theories have been advanced as to why we have sinuses and just what they are supposed to do. Of course, we know what happens when something goes wrong with the sinuses—we develop the symptoms of sinusitis. But what is the function of this part of the anatomy in a healthy, disease-free individual? Why do we have sinuses in the first place?

Scientists have been trying to unravel the mysteries of the sinuses for centuries. Around 400 B.C., Hippocrates speculated that they played a role in draining mucus from the brain to the nasal cavity. Ancient Indian scripts and the Talmud first suggested that the sinuses might be linked with disease, although the exact reasons weren't known. In the fifteenth century, Leonardo da Vinci studied sinus anatomy, and even sketched pictures of the maxillary and frontal cavities.

Despite all this scrutiny, what continues to baffle scientists even today is that although the sinuses have a number of different jobs in the human body, none appear obvious or essential. For instance, hollow spaces make the dense skull lighter, which may hold some advantage. Sinuses also offer some protection from trauma by acting as a kind of shock absorber. They add resonance to the voice, contribute in minor ways to our sense of smell, and may enhance immune system mechanisms. Mucus produced by the sinuses warms and moistens the air, and helps trap small airborne particles and bacteria. On the other hand, the nose also produces mucus (and much more of it) that performs the same function.

In recent years, researchers have hypothesized that the explanation for sinus oddities is that although we now walk on our own two feet, we have inherited the sinus anatomy of four-legged animals. They point out as evidence of this the fact that in defiance of all logic, the maxillary and sphenoid ostia are located at the top rather than the bottom of those sinuses, rendering drainage difficult and increasing the likelihood of blockage. But whatever the answer turns out to be, it is clear that although the sinuses may play only bit parts in the normal functioning of the human body, they play a leading role in sinus disease.

A VULNERABILITY TO INFLAMMATION AND OBSTRUCTION

Now that you have a better grasp of the structure and function of your sinuses, it's easy to see how vulnerable they can be to inflammation and obstruction. In the next two chapters, we'll explore how problems ranging from colds and allergies to air pollution and compromised immunity can impair the sinuses and lead to sinusitis.

CHAPTER 3

Respiratory Infections, Allergies, and Asthma

It's really not all that surprising that people confuse colds and allergies with sinusitis. Acute sinusitis most commonly follows an upper respiratory infection (URI), and repeated colds and allergies can lead to chronic sinusitis. Over the course of the last few decades, allergies and asthma have become more common worldwide, most likely due to a corresponding increase in urban air pollution. This is clearly a major contributing factor to the rise in sinusitis. In this chapter, we'll explore the links between each of these ailments and sinus disease: how they are similar, but also what key distinctions exist among them.

RESPIRATORY INFECTIONS AND SINUSITIS

Viral respiratory infections—that is, colds and influenza (flu)—comprise the single most common predisposing factor for sinusitis. Respiratory viruses are generally airborne and enter the body through the nose, mouth, and lungs. The respiratory tract offers a large and vulnerable area of attack for an airborne virus, which can invade the body through microscopic breaks in delicate mucous membranes. Most often, URIs are spread by fairly direct contact—such as when children share toys or when a person next to you coughs or sneezes without covering his or her mouth—but occasionally you may be infected by moisture droplets circulating through a confined area such as a plane, train, or bus. Adults have on average two to three colds each year, while children experience three to eight or even more.

All About Colds

Physicians refer to the common cold as viral rhinitis—that is, an inflammatory condition of the nose that is caused by a virus. Colds are passed from person to person by sneezing, coughing, personal contact, and touching objects contaminated by a cold virus. Anything from stress and depression to smoking and a lack of sleep can increase your susceptibility to colds—in fact, the risk of rhinitis is double for children who live in damp houses and have parents who smoke. But a virus must actually enter the respiratory tract for a person to get sick. As we grow older, we contract fewer infections because we gradually build up immunity to many cold-causing viruses. Although many different viruses can cause colds, about half are due to the human rhinovirus.

Symptoms of a Cold

You know you're coming down with a cold when you experience symptoms such as a sore throat and a runny or stuffy nose. The first sign of a cold is often a feeling of dryness, itchiness, or irritation at the back of the nose or throat, or on the roof of the mouth. In the next day or two, a variety of other symptoms may develop, including:

- Congestion
- Thin, watery discharge that may or may not turn thick and greenish yellow
- Tickle in the throat
- Sore throat
- Hoarseness
- Sneezing
- Cough
- Low-grade fever
- Headache
- Muscle aches
- Fatigue
- Watery, red eyes

- Loss of appetite
- A general feeling of illness or malaise
- Swollen lymph nodes in the neck
- Cold sores

Treating a Cold

There is no medicine to cure a common cold. However, if you are particularly susceptible to sinusitis, especially following colds, your doctor may recommend treatment such as oral decongestants to reduce membrane swelling within the nose and sinus cavity. By relieving sinus blockage, decongestants may help prevent the development of secondary sinus disease. Otherwise, unless symptoms are persistent or severe, or if they aggravate an existing respiratory condition, it is not usually necessary to see your physician. A common cold usually runs its course within ten days. During this time, you can lessen your discomfort by practicing simple home care. For example, get plenty of rest; don't smoke; drink clear liquids; cut back on heavy foods, alcohol, and caffeine; use humidifiers or steam treatments; and take over-the-counter medication to relieve discomfort.

Cold Medications

Over-the-counter remedies such as analgesics and decongestants can relieve some uncomfortable upper respiratory symptoms. However, they have no impact on the virus and do not shorten the duration of a cold. They can also be improperly used. For example, steer clear of remedies that include antihistamines, which are meant to treat allergies, not colds. In addition to antihistamines, there are basically four other types of drugs used in cold and cough preparations: decongestants, analgesics, cough suppressants, and expectorants. Decongestants allow you to breathe freely and, because they shrink swollen nasal membranes, even offer some protection against secondary sinus infection. Analgesics control fever and offer pain relief; the cough suppressant dextromethorphan (by far the most commonly used drug of this type) suppresses irritating, unproductive coughs, without interfering with useful productive coughs that clear phlegm; expectorants such as guaifenesin loosen phlegm and help the cough lift it out of bronchial tubes. Dextromethorphan and guaifenesin have few side effects, but decongestants and analgesics can both cause a number of adverse reactions and are not for everyone. (Read about cold medications in greater detail in chapter 6.)

A Special Word About the Flu

The flu—or influenza—is a viral infection that causes more severe symptoms than an ordinary cold, notably fever, headache, muscle aches, and weakness. And while influenza itself is bad enough, its complications can be even worse. The flu can lead to sinus, ear, and bronchial infections, as well as potentially life-threatening pneumonia and Reye's syndrome. Reye's syndrome is a rare condition in children and adolescents that involves brain swelling and liver failure; it has been linked to the use of aspirin during influenza, which is the reason why you should never give aspirin to children.

The Three Flu Viruses

There are three types of influenza virus: Types A, B, and C. Type A—the most common—regularly develops new strains and is responsible for a new epidemic every few years. In North America, flu season generally begins in November and lasts through March. Types B and C are more stable viruses. Type B causes only small outbreaks, while the symptoms of Type C resemble those of the common cold. Any one of these three flu viruses can infect you when you inhale contaminated moisture droplets from the air.

Symptoms of the Flu

Unlike colds, which tend to come on gradually, flu symptoms often descend quickly and dramatically. One minute you feel fine, and the next you are feverish and dizzy and have an overall sense of unwellness. In addition to cold symptoms such as a stuffy nose and sore throat, flu sufferers commonly endure headaches, muscle aches, fever, and chills. Other symptoms may include a nagging cough, hoarseness, laryngitis, nasal discharge, sweating, fatigue, clammy skin, nosebleeds, nausea, vomiting, diarrhea, joint pain, and loss of appetite. Sneezing, a common symptom when you have a cold, is not usually seen with the flu. Also unlike colds, the flu is—at least at first—concentrated in the lower respiratory system. As it enters the lungs, it initially causes a dry cough, but this is often followed in two or three days by a wet, productive cough. When a persistent cough is accompanied by chest pain and a high fever, pneumonia should be suspected (especially in older people).

Who Is at Risk?

In a healthy person, flu symptoms normally run their course in seven to ten days. However, certain people are at greater risk for severe flu symptoms and their complications. These include the elderly, those with impaired immune systems, and people who have chronic medical problems. Each year the Centers for Disease Control and Prevention (CDC) issue new guidelines, establishing an immunization schedule that calls for people at the greatest risk for complications to be vaccinated first.

WHO NEEDS A FLU SHOT?

According to the CDC, those in most need of flu shots generally include:

- People over the age of sixty-five. As we grow older, our ability to combat infection wanes, making us more susceptible to complications ranging from sinusitis to pneumonia.
- People with chronic medical conditions, such as heart disease; lung problems, such as asthma; liver or kidney disease; diabetes; chronic anemia; leukemia and lymphoma; HIV infection and AIDS.
- People who are taking immunosuppressive drugs, including chemotherapy or radiation for cancer; drugs to prevent rejection of organ transplants; and corticosteroids for conditions such as ulcerative colitis or arthritis.
- Women who will be in the second or third trimester of pregnancy during flu season.
- Health workers who care for high-risk patients.

Prevention Is Key

Vaccines are made anew each year to combat the flu strains most likely to cause disease in the coming winter. The priority is to immunize those at highest risk first, because vaccine availability varies from year to year. Of course, if more vaccine is available, anyone of any age can benefit from immunization. Flu shots are 60 to 70 percent effective in preventing influenza.

A few people should not receive flu shots. Because the virus for the vaccine is grown in chicken embryos, this includes anyone who is allergic to eggs, as well as those who had an allergic reaction to a previous flu shot. A typical reaction is local inflammation, and some people also experience mild flu symptoms. However, it is a myth that flu shots give you the flu—the vaccine is made from killed virus that cannot multiply in the body, so this is impossible.

For people who fail to get the vaccine, there are several prescription medications that can prevent the flu or at least reduce the severity of its symptoms. These include amantadine and rimantadine, which are effective against the Type A virus. Two drugs—oseltamivir and zanamivir—reduce the symptoms of both Type A and Type B influenza. Of course, simple measures—such as frequent handwashing and making sure people cover their mouths when they cough or sneeze—are effective in preventing the flu as well as colds.

Diagnosis and Treatment

Doctors generally diagnose influenza according to your symptoms. A physical examination may confirm diagnosis, and tests such as nose and throat cultures will rule out other possible causes of symptoms, such as sinusitis or strep throat. Because there is no cure for the flu, the goal of treatment is to relieve symptoms. Home care is much the same as for a cold. When you have a fever, it is especially important to drink plenty of fluids, such as water and juice. Having enough liquids also keeps mucus thin and easier to expel from the body. Take acetaminophen (Tylenol) or NSAIDs (nonsteroidal anti-inflammatory drugs such as Advil or Motrin) to relieve muscle aches and pains; because of the risk of Reye's syndrome, never give children or adolescents aspirin for the flu. Decongestants relieve congestion and may even help prevent secondary sinus and ear infections. Cough suppressants can also be safely used. Antihistamines are recommended only when there is an allergic component to your illness; otherwise, they may cause significant drowsiness, and their drying effects thicken mucus and can lead to further sinus blockage. Antibiotics are inappropriate for influenza and other viral infections. If you are elderly, have a chronic disease, or are otherwise at risk, ask your doctor about antiviral medications such as amantadine.

The Link Between Upper Respiratory Infections and Sinusitis

When a cold or flu virus attacks the upper respiratory system, the sinuses are nearly always involved. In most cases, this means mild inflammation and swelling of the mucous membranes, an increase in mucous secretions, and sometimes a tightening or sensation of sinus pressure around the face. When you first come down with an upper respiratory infection, symptoms such as headache, fever, and congestion are generally due to the cold or flu virus invading your body—not to sinusitis. In fact, any symptoms of sinusitis are at first overshadowed by acute URI symptoms. As the virus runs its course, there is no certain way to prevent the subsequent development of sinus disease. But if the sinuses continue to remain open and drain freely, theoretically they, too, will recover within the ten days of infection.

How URIs Promote Sinusitis

Researchers aren't certain of all the exact mechanisms by which URIs promote sinusitis, but it appears that the inflammatory response to a virus leads to a decreased oxygen supply and temporary ciliary defects. You may recall that cilia are the microscopic hairs that line the respiratory passages and play a vital role in moving along the overlying mucous blanket. Good mucociliary clearance is essential to clearing mucus from the respiratory tract and keeping the sinuses healthy. However, a viral infection of the upper respiratory system causes inflammation of the mucous membranes that line the nose, throat, sinuses, ears, windpipe, and voice box. This inflammatory response can eventually close the sinuses, making the capillary bed the only available source of oxygen. In consequence, leukocytes rush into the area and lead to the secretion of the enzymes elastase and collagenase, which destroy cells and inhibit ciliary movement. The influenza virus infects the most cells and causes the greatest cell destruction.

ALLERGIES AND SINUSITIS

The connection between allergies and sinusitis is less well established than the link between URIs and sinus disease. Nonetheless, the evidence clearly supports allergies as a major risk factor for sinusitis. Research has shown that more than half of all children with allergies have abnormalities in their sinuses. Likewise, another study revealed that more than half of chronic sinusitis sufferers had positive skin tests, meaning that they had allergies.

In order to prevent sinus problems, allergies must be strictly controlled. When you have a sinus infection and an allergic reaction at the same time, both conditions need to be correctly diagnosed and treated. Certain substances, called allergens, are responsible for allergic reactions in susceptible individuals. Good management of allergies consists of identifying and avoiding allergens, and often medical treatment such as antihistamines and immunotherapy.

Are You Allergy-Prone?

The tendency to have allergic reactions—which is known as atopy—
is genetic, or inherited. However, it is the allergic tendency—not specific allergies—that is passed on. For example, while your mother
may have had hay fever (a respiratory problem), you may have
eczema (a skin problem). Atopic individuals are born with a predisposition to manufacture large amounts of antibodies known as
immunoglobulin E (IgE). When you are atopic, exposure to an allergen stimulates the production of IgE. If the allergen and specific IgE
for the allergen link together, mast cells are directed to discharge substances that bring on allergic symptoms.

An Allergic Reaction

Allergic reactions, and the exact mechanisms of the immune system
that cause them, are not completely understood. However, we do
know that when a foreign protein enters the body, the immune system sometimes mistakenly reacts to it—even when the protein itself is
causing little or no harm. While the immune system normally protects us from dangerous disease-causing microorganisms, when you
have allergies, it "protects" you from benign substances. This inappropriate reaction leads to swollen nasal membranes, sinus headaches, rashes, itches, and other unpleasant reactions familiar to all
allergy sufferers.

In an atopic, or allergy-prone, person, the onset of an allergy takes
place when antigen-presenting cells are first exposed to a potential
antigen (an allergy-provoking substance), such as house dust, pollen,
animal dander, or mold. If the person's body perceives this substance
to be an invader, the antigen-presenting cells activate other cells to
produce an unusually large amount of IgE antibodies. During this initial exposure, IgE molecules attach to mast cells. Inside mast cells are
granules that contain a variety of protective chemicals, the most well-
known of which is histamine.

The initial exposure does not lead to an allergic reaction. It is
repeated exposure or sensitization to the substance that causes allergies to develop. When sensitized mast cells are next exposed to the
substance, IgE antibodies on the mast cells bind to it, and the cells
release their histamine and other mediators of inflammation. These
mediators cause symptoms such as itching, sneezing, congestion, and
increased production of mucus. Two to eight hours later, there is an

additional response, which is known as a late-phase reaction. It is associated with an accumulation of various kinds of inflammatory cells in the nose, a buildup that causes increased sensitivity to allergy-provoking substances and even nonallergic irritants.

CELLS INVOLVED IN ALLERGIC REACTIONS

A number of different cells produced in the bone marrow contribute to allergic reactions:

- **Mast cells,** the tissue form of basophils, are important in a variety of conditions such as allergy, inflammation, tissue remodeling, responses to parasite infestation, and angiogenesis (the creation of blood vessels).
- **Eosinophils, basophils, neutrophils,** and **monocytes** are also important in allergic reactions. Scientists are currently focusing increased attention on the role that eosinophils play in chronic sinusitis. When eosinophils enter tissue, inflammatory substances such as cytokines and chemical mediators are released. These reactions cause tissue damage such as increased sodium absorption and consequent swelling. Eosinophilia—high levels of eosinophils—is also associated with asthma and nasal polyps.

The Triggers of Respiratory Allergies

Allergens can enter our bodies through the airways, skin, gastrointestinal tract, or circulatory system. Naturally, when you are prone to sinusitis, concern focuses on airborne allergens that enter through the nose or mouth. These include substances such as household dust and dust mites, mold spores, animal dander, and pollen. It is airborne allergens that are responsible for the frequent sneezing, runny nose, stuffiness, and red, itchy, watery eyes typical of allergic rhinitis. Often there is also a postnasal drip that causes a scratchy or irritated throat. Seasonal allergic rhinitis, or hay fever, occurs at certain times of the year, when grass, weed, or tree pollen thrives. Some people experience symptoms year-round due to allergens such as the saliva, excretions, and body parts of dust mites and cockroaches. In addition to their role in allergic rhinitis, airborne allergens can trigger or worsen the symptoms of sinusitis; affect the lining of the lungs and cause asthmatic episodes; or inflame the conjunctiva of the eye, leading to pinkeye (conjunctivitis).

COMMON AIRBORNE ALLERGENS

The most common airborne allergens are:

Plant pollens
Animal dander and fur
House dust
House dust mites and cockroaches
Mold spores
Cigarette smoke
Cleaners
Solvents

Diagnosing Allergies

Allergies are often diagnosed by your physician through a detailed medical history and physical examination. To verify the diagnosis and determine which allergens are the ones that affect you, you may be sent to a board-certified allergist or other qualified allergy specialist (such as an otolaryngologist) for further testing. In prick tests or patch tests, your skin is exposed to small amounts of allergens. If you do have an allergy to a particular substance, the skin around that area will redden and a small welt will form. This means that the IgE antibodies specific to the allergen have responded by triggering the release of histamine. An alternative to skin testing is a blood test known as RAST (Radioallergosorbent Test); this measures the level of allergen-specific IgE antibodies in the blood.

Avoiding Allergens

Treatment of allergies entails elimination or avoidance of the offending allergens, and in many cases additional medical treatment. Once the triggers of your symptoms have been identified, it's time to make some lifestyle changes in an effort to steer clear of them. One of the best ways you can control allergies is to exert control over your environment. Although removing allergens can present a challenge, when you minimize your exposure to the stimuli that provoke allergic reactions, you get the added benefit of reducing your need for medication.

There are many simple, practical steps you can take to eliminate dust mites, mold, animal dander, smoke, pollen, and other common allergens from your surroundings. For example, it is important to clean your home—or have it cleaned—on a regular basis. Many people find it helpful to use "green" products, which are safe and natural alternatives to harsh chemicals. Stress to your family and friends that your home is a smoke-free environment, and if you have pets, at least ban them from the bedroom. If your allergies are seasonal, close the windows and use air-conditioning during pollen season. Also avoid engaging in strenuous outdoor activities when the pollen count is high. (Turn to chapter 9 for more tips on avoiding allergens and allergy-proofing your home.)

Allergy Medications

When the avoidance of allergens alone is insufficient to control your allergies, rest assured that a plethora of prescription and over-the-counter medications awaits you. However, because many of these drugs have side effects, it is best to consult with your physician before using even over-the-counter remedies. Foremost among allergy medications are antihistamines, which block the histamine receptors on nasal tissue. This helps control inflammation and swelling, and reduces allergic reactions such as increased production of mucus and general irritation. Keep in mind, though, that antihistamines can have a number of side effects, ranging from nervousness and insomnia in some people to drowsiness in others. Newer, nondrowsy antihistamines are also available by prescription.

Other medications for allergies include decongestants, cromolyn sodium, steroids, and immunotherapy. By constricting blood vessels and thus shrinking swollen membranes, decongestants help counteract the effects of histamine. But these drugs, too, have side effects, including nervousness, dizziness, rapid heart rate, and insomnia. Consequently, decongestants should be used with care in people with high blood pressure. Cromolyn sodium is a safe, over-the-counter nasal spray that inhibits the release of histamine from mast cells. It has few if any side effects, but must be used for two to three weeks before it takes effect. Corticosteroid tablets are powerful anti-inflammatory medications that reduce swelling and inflammation of mucous membranes. These drugs can be enormously beneficial but must be used with extreme care due to serious side effects that range from bloating, weight gain, and stomach upset to an increased risk of serious health problems such as osteoporosis, hypertension, and cataracts. The topical forms of corticosteroids (i.e., intranasal and inhaled by mouth) are safer than pills or capsules that you swallow. Finally, immunotherapy is helpful to some—although not all—allergy sufferers. Immunotherapy consists of a series of allergy or desensitizing shots. It carries a small but significant risk of anaphylaxis, a life-threatening allergic reaction involving a sharp drop in blood pressure and difficulty breathing. (Read in greater detail about allergy medications in chapter 6.)

The Link Between Allergies and Sinusitis

As with upper respiratory infections, the exact mechanism by which allergic disease leads to sinusitis remains unclear. Most likely, nasal inflammation brought on by allergies leads to blockage of the vital osteomeatal unit (OMU), the shared area into which the maxillary, frontal, and anterior ethmoid sinuses all drain. OMU obstruction, in turn, can provoke secondary bacterial infection.

Allergic Mucous Membranes Are More Vulnerable

The mucous membranes of people with allergies appear to be more susceptible to infection because of the presence of cells called eosinophils. These cells release mediators such as major basic protein, which has toxic effects on the cilia and on the mucosal surface. In support of this theory, doctors typically find tissue eosinophilia in children with chronic sinusitis who require surgery. This is also true in those who suffer from asthma. In addition, researchers have noted a connection between the severity of sinus disease and IgE levels, leading them to believe that the inflammatory responses in sinusitis and asthma may be similar. A hypothesis is that chronic sinusitis may be a disease of atopic immune activation.

ASTHMA AND SINUSITIS

People with sinus problems are more likely than others to also suffer from asthma, an increasingly common disease in the United States. Fortunately, the treatment of asthma has improved dramatically in recent years, and today this chronic lung ailment is an almost entirely controllable disease. Doctors have discovered that using anti-inflammatory drugs regularly, even when symptoms are not present, significantly reduces inflammation and hyperreactivity of airways in the lungs. Studies have also revealed that good medical management of sinusitis results in improvement in asthma symptoms.

All About Asthma

Asthma is a disease of the lungs characterized by chronic inflammation and reversible blockage of the airways. Its most common symptoms are wheezing, coughing, chest tightness, and shortness of breath. When you have asthma, you have hyperreactive, or twitchy, airways. This means that your airways are sensitive to triggers such as allergens, upper respiratory infections, environmental pollutants, cold air, and exercise. But the triggers of symptoms vary from person to person, and the cold air that brings on an asthmatic episode in one person may have no effect at all on another.

An Asthmatic Episode

When you experience an asthmatic attack, or episode, three major events take place inside your lungs to block the flow of air through them:

- An inflammatory response directs a variety of cells into the lung's bronchial tubes, which can thicken their inside walls and lead to blockages.
- The bronchial tubes are surrounded by bands of smooth muscles that are hyperreactive, or twitchy. When triggered, the muscles tighten around the airways in an attempt to expel what they perceive to be hostile invaders. This further narrows air passages and reduces the flow of air through them.
- Glands inside the airways clog already narrowed passages with the excretion of excessive amounts of thick, sticky mucus.

Diagnosing Asthma

An accurate diagnosis of asthma entails a detailed medical history and a thorough physical examination. As with allergies, your medical history is of special importance, because linking triggers and symptoms is vital to controlling as well as diagnosing the disease. Another key aspect is objective measurement of lung function. Assessments of breathing called spirometry, or pulmonary function tests, measure the level of airflow obstruction in the lungs. Spirometry can usually be conducted in your physician's office. Other tests your doctor may order include chest or sinus X rays, or other imaging studies; a complete blood count (CBC); allergy tests; bronchial provocation testing (to measure your sensitivity to suspected triggers); and an exercise challenge (when exercise is a suspected trigger of symptoms).

Asthma Varies in Severity

Some people who have asthma experience only occasional wheezing, from which they recover spontaneously or with the aid of a bronchodilator (a medication that relieves constriction of the airways). Others have severe attacks that are unresponsive to inhaled medication. Some attacks are preceded by sinus or nasal symptoms, or a productive cough. Types of asthma include:

- *Mild Intermittent*: Symptoms include occasional episodes of wheezing from which you recover spontaneously or with the aid of a bronchodilator. Diagnosis is usually made through medical history.
- *Moderate Intermittent*: In this type of asthma, episodes are still occasional, but can require more treatment. Exercise may trigger attacks. Diagnosis involves using a simple home monitoring device called a peak flow meter, which measures your maximum rate of expiratory flow in liters per minute. Keeping a chart of this measurement over a period of weeks can give your physician information about any major day-to-day changes and the times when attacks are most apt to occur (such as at night or early in the morning, or following exercise).
- *Mild Persistent*: Symptoms occur several times a week, frequently after exercise. However, they are easily reversed. Diagnosis is made through peak flow monitoring, an evaluation of causes, a chest X ray, and spirometry (an assessment of your breathing).
- *Moderate Persistent*: This form of asthma requires regular treatment. Symptoms occur frequently, and may be severe. Exercise is often a trigger. Your physician will carefully evaluate the causes of the increasing severity of your symptoms.
- *Severe Persistent*: Persistent symptoms require continuous treatment, which may include visits to the emergency room and/or hospitalization. Your doctor will conduct tests such as spirometry, DLCO (diffusion capacity of the lung for carbon monoxide), and sinus CT scanning. He or she will reevaluate underlying causes such as sinus disease, fungal infection, and aspirin sensitivity.

Managing Asthma

Asthma treatment typically involves steering clear of triggers and taking medication. Again there are similarities to allergies, because it is essential to make changes in your environment in order to avoid, when possible, the triggers of your symptoms. But there are also notable differences: some of the triggers of asthma—such as cold air or exercise—are either unavoidable or not desirable to avoid. But if you take medication before going out on a chilly winter night or playing a game of tennis, there is usually no problem. Depending on the frequency and severity of your symptoms, your physician will recommend that you take medications routinely or on an as-needed basis. There are two types of asthma medications: anti-inflammatory drugs and bronchodilators. Anti-inflammatory medications are taken to prevent the symptoms of asthma, while bronchodilators are used to control symptoms once they occur. (Read more about asthma medications in chapter 6.)

The Link Between Asthma and Sinusitis

At least half the people who are treated for asthma also experience sinus or nasal symptoms of some kind. The symptoms are often allergic and may be triggered by factors such as dampness, mold, animal dander, pests, or pollen. The chronic nasal inflammation of sinus disease is another common trigger of asthma symptoms. But as with upper respiratory infections and allergies, scientists have yet to pin down the exact mechanism that explains how sinusitis causes asthma. One distinct probability is that postnasal drip into the lower airways leads to increased inflammation and hyperreactivity. Asthma may also be aggravated if the nasal obstruction makes you breathe through your mouth, causing a loss of heat and moisture in the lower airways. Whatever the exact connection turns out to be, one thing is clear: controlling sinusitis can lead to significant improvements in the management of asthma. As a result, if you successfully manage your sinus disease, you will not have to take as much asthma medication as those who do not.

OTHER COMMON CAUSES OF SINUSITIS

Although upper respiratory infections and allergies account for most cases of sinusitis, many different factors can contribute to this

ASTHMA, NASAL POLYPS, SINUSITIS, AND ASPIRIN INTOLERANCE

Many asthma sufferers are sensitive to aspirin. But it is especially important to avoid aspirin and aspirin products if you suffer from Samter's syndrome, whose three components are asthma, nasal polyps, and aspirin intolerance. This condition can also involve an increased population of eosinophils. Under these circumstances, taking aspirin can bring on sudden and severe breathing problems.

condition. In the next chapter, we'll explore other common causes of sinusitis, including swollen adenoids, anatomic variations, cystic fibrosis, air pollution, and immune problems.

CHAPTER 4

Other Common Causes of Sinusitis

In addition to colds, allergies, and asthma, many other factors play a significant role in sinusitis. As we mentioned earlier, sinusitis is rarely due to one single cause. Instead, physicians describe it as multifactorial because so many different factors combine to make you susceptible to this disease. Some—such as nasal polyps and cystic fibrosis—have long been recognized for the parts they play. Others—including immune impairment, air pollution, and fungi—have captured the attention of researchers and scientists in more recent years,

MORE CONTRIBUTING FACTORS TO SINUSITIS

- Nasal obstruction due to conditions such as swollen adenoids, nasal polyps, prior surgery, foreign bodies, and tumors
- Anatomic variations, including cleft palate, concha bullosa, and deviated septum
- Underlying disease, such as cystic fibrosis or ciliary dyskinesia
- Dental infection
- Air pollution (outdoor and indoor)
- Barotrauma—injuries due to changes in ambient pressure—resulting from activities such as air travel or scuba diving
- Immune problems, which may be congenital or acquired
- Fungal infection (noninvasive and invasive)

as they seek to understand why sinusitis has become so increasingly widespread. In this chapter, we discuss these and other common causes of sinus disease.

NASAL OBSTRUCTION

Sinusitis is invariably associated with some form of nasal obstruction. This obstruction can be the result of inflammation (such as following an upper respiratory infection or allergic reaction), or it can be mechanical in nature. In this section, we discuss some prominent mechanical causes of obstruction.

Adenoids

These clusters of tissue at the back of the nose and throat have long been known to play a role in otitis media (middle-ear infections), and now it is clear that they also contribute to sinus disease in one of two ways. When they become enlarged, adenoids obstruct airflow and cause the retention of secretions. This in turn can lead to infection. Alternatively, the adenoids themselves and nearby tonsils may become infected, and this infection can spread directly to the sinuses. In children who suffer from chronic sinusitis or recurrent acute attacks, it may be beneficial to remove the adenoids. Adults are less likely to be affected by adenoid problems.

Nasal Polyps

Polyps are rounded, grapelike tissue growths that form on mucous membranes in various locations throughout the body. Because you may have heard more about polyps that develop in the colon, initially you may feel nervous if your physician suspects that you have nasal polyps. However, while intestinal polyps often become malignant, polyps that develop in the nose and sinuses generally retain the same cellular structure as normal mucosal tissue and thus remain benign.

The Causes of Nasal Polyps

Nasal polyps are not a disease in and of themselves. Instead, they are a physical manifestation that may be an end result of a number of different disease processes, only one of which is sinusitis. These include:

- Chronic sinusitis
- Allergies
- Allergic fungal sinusitis
- Cystic fibrosis

NASAL POLYPS MAY HAVE A GENETIC BASIS

- Cystic fibrosis is an autosomal-recessive disorder that is frequently associated with nasal polyps. It is caused by a genetic abnormality.
- Woakes' syndrome is a rare autosomal-recessive disorder of bony nasal deformation associated with recurrent bilateral nasal polyposis (multiple polyps on both sides of the nose).
- Nasal polyposis in association with asthma and aspirin intolerance is known as Samter's syndrome, ASA triad, or aspirin-sensitive asthma. Clusters of this disorder in families suggest that it has a genetic basis.

Nasal Polyps Vary in Severity

Because they have so many different causes, nasal polyps vary widely in severity. People who develop this problem generally fall into two groups: those who have general respiratory disease and those who experience solely nasal disease. When they are a result of general respiratory disease, polyps are more difficult to treat and contain.

Many nasal polyps occur as single, localized problems and cause no significant difficulties. Others cause massive mucosal changes and actually lead to facial deformity. Sometimes even a small growth restricts a nasal passage, slowing drainage and allowing infection to develop. A single polyp can also lead to the generation of multiple polyps, or grow so large that it protrudes into the osteomeatal unit (OMU) of the nasal cavity. When a polyp reduces ventilation in the meatus and the ethmoid cells, it creates an environment favorable to the development of additional polyps.

Key Characteristics of Nasal Polyp Development

- *Eosinophilia*: This inflammatory response involves the release of important mediators of inflammation by white blood cells called eosinophils. On the plus side, these mediators play an important role in the elimination of parasites. However, they also cause damaging inflammation in the sinus membranes.

- *Swelling*: Mediators cause various types of tissue damage in the sinuses. For instance, one mediator increases sodium absorption, and a high tissue salt content results in water absorption and subsequent swelling.

- *Changes in the regrowth of injured mucous membranes*: Abnormal cell changes occur when the injured mucous membranes of nasal polyps attempt to regenerate. For example, goblet cells may come to replace most of the normal sinus tissue, resulting in a significant increase in mucous production.

- *The development of new, abnormal glands*: Nasal polyps encourage the growth of large, distorted glands that are completely different from normal glands in the nose and sinuses.

More Causes of Mechanical Obstruction

In addition to adenoids and polyps, a variety of other forms of mechanical obstruction may factor into sinus disease. For example, excessive scarring generated by prior disease, fractures, or surgery can lead to obstruction. At times, sinusitis develops in response to a foreign body that somehow becomes lodged in the nose. Not surprisingly, this occurrence is most frequent in children. In critical-care units within hospitals, special care must be taken with patients who require nasogastric or nasotracheal tubes; the longer a tube must be left in, the greater chance a patient has of developing sinusitis. A tumor is another relatively uncommon but still possible basis for obstruction.

ANATOMIC VARIATIONS

Anatomic variations also play a key role in sinusitis. However, some researchers believe that their size rather than their mere presence predisposes a person toward obstruction, inflammation, and infection. For example, large concha bullosae (deformities of middle turbinates in the nose) are more likely than small ones to cause inflammatory sinus disease. Other variations in nose or sinus anatomy—such as a congenital malformation—may also be implicated. For example, children born with choanal atresia (a bony or membranous partition across the back of the nose) or a cleft palate experience an unusually high number of both middle-ear infections and sinusitis. In this section, we look at several of the more common anatomic variations that contribute to sinus disease.

Cleft Palate

This congenital malformation is characterized by a gap in the roof of the mouth, often accompanied by a cleft lip. Children born with a cleft palate experience difficulties with breathing, eating, and speech development. Other problems, such as sinus and ear infections, are also common. This is because the palate normally separates and protects the nose from the mouth, especially when a child eats and drinks. When there is no separation, the mucous membranes are continually irritated and inflamed, setting the stage for infection. Even though most cleft palates are surgically corrected by the age of two, many children with this malformation have already developed chronic sinusitis by that time.

Deviated Septum

In normal anatomy, the nasal septum (the wall between the nostrils) is never totally straight. But if you have a significantly deviated septum, the soft and bony portions of the septum are badly crooked or bowed. This condition may restrict or block nasal passages, creating an environment hospitable to infection. In medical terms, a deviated septum can compress the middle turbinate and compromise the middle meatus. It can also make breathing difficult. When this anatomic variation generates problems, it can be surgically straightened. However, in many cases, even a significantly deviated septum does not cause noticeable difficulties.

Concha Bullosa

This deformity of the middle turbinate in the nose is a somewhat controversial cause of sinusitis. In this condition, the middle turbinate becomes distended by a large hollow space (concha bullosa) within its bony core. Medically speaking, this means that an aerated middle turbinate occurs when ethmoid cells grow larger than usual and pneumatize the area. The resulting compression of the uncinate process and obstruction of the middle meatus and infundibulum form the basis for recurrent inflammatory sinus disease. However, many physicians believe that concha bullosae—even large ones—do not inevitably lead to sinusitis. The key seems to lie in whether or not there is contact between the concha and the lateral nasal wall. This is because as long as there is an open space, the mucus can flow freely.

It is the bony wall of the concha that causes the compression and obstruction by contacting the adjacent lateral wall.

UNDERLYING DISEASE

In some cases, the root cause of sinusitis is a systemic disease such as cystic fibrosis. It is essential to manage any underlying illness in order to successfully treat and control sinusitis.

Cystic Fibrosis

A relatively common genetic disorder, cystic fibrosis (CF) is characterized by persistent lung infections along with an inability to absorb fats and other nutrients from food. It is caused by a genetic abnormality. Before the era of modern medicine, children with this disease lived only into their teens. With today's improved standards of care, life expectancy extends into the twenties and thirties.

Thick, syrupy mucus is a hallmark symptom of cystic fibrosis. In fact, the mucus of children with CF is thirty to sixty times more viscous than normal mucus. This leads to lung infection, blockage, and damage, exemplified by symptoms such as wheezing and coughing. Since the ability to digest food is impaired, affected children may also suffer from chronic diarrhea. Even if they have a good appetite, they may fail to gain weight.

In the nose and sinuses, cystic fibrosis commonly leads to chronic nasal obstruction, nasal polyps, and sinusitis. (Nasal polyps are otherwise an unusual phenomenon in children.) Although the cilia are not directly affected by CF, the extreme thickness of mucus makes it difficult for these tiny hairs to successfully propel the mucous blanket forward. Consequent obstruction creates an environment of decreased oxygen and increased toxins, which causes ciliary damage, swelling, and further inflammation.

Ciliary Diseases

Mucociliary clearance—the normal production and flow of mucus around the nasal passages and sinuses—is essential to the proper functioning of the sinuses. The beating of tiny cilia helps to sweep the mucous blanket through the sinus cavities. In order to successfully accomplish this movement, the cilia and the mucous blanket must work together as a unit. The beating motion of cilia in the mucous blanket's inner layer propels the outer thicker, viscous layer forward through the sinuses.

Many factors can impair the normal functioning of the cilia. These include viruses, decreased oxygen availability, changes in temperature, dehydration, environmental irritants, chemicals, and drugs. Primary ciliary dyskinesia (PCD) is a term used to refer to diseases characterized by structural abnormalities in the cilia; in immotile cilia syndrome, there is a total lack of movement of cilia. A rare genetic disorder known as Kartagener's syndrome is a type of PCD. This disease involves situs inversus (in which the location of body organs is inverted or transposed), bronchiectasis (the distortion or enlargement of one or more of the bronchial tubes in the lungs), infertility (in males), and sinusitis. In a PCD-related condition called ciliary disorientation, the cilia are normal in structure and beat, but the beat's direction is disoriented. This problem is seen in some cases of maxillary chronic sinusitis.

Gastroesophageal Reflux Disease

Nearly one out of three Americans suffers from this problem, which is also known as reflux, acid reflux, esophagitis, or GERD. Reflux is the backward flow of acid from the stomach up into the esophagus. Heartburn, the most prevalent symptom, is a burning sensation in the upper abdomen or chest that occurs when a person with this disorder eats, bends, or lies down. Reflux is especially common at night (particularly when you stretch out after a heavy meal) and most frequently affects older people and pregnant women. In some cases, stomach acid backs up all the way into the nose. When this happens, you may notice a bitter or sour taste in the back of your mouth and throat, followed by a burning in the nose. If it occurs on a consistent basis, and the stomach contents cause continual irritation and inflammation of the mucous membranes, sinusitis can develop.

Reflux arises when there is a leak in the opening (or hiatus) at the junction of the esophagus and stomach. This leak is more likely to occur when the lower esophageal sphincter (LES) muscle at the base of the esophagus grows weak. Greasy or fatty foods, chocolate, and alcohol may contribute to weakening of the LES muscle. But whatever its underlying cause may be, persistent reflux can lead to inflammation and chronic sinusitis.

DENTAL INFECTION

Bacteria associated with a dental infection can also invade the sinuses. Dental problems are most frequently associated with infections of the maxillary sinuses, which are located right above the posterior upper teeth in the cheekbones. If a stubborn case of maxillary sinusitis resists other forms of treatment, your physician may advise you to consult a dentist to determine whether a chronically infected or broken-off upper tooth is at the core of the problem. When this is the case, dental surgery may be required to eliminate the underlying cause of sinus infection. In addition, whenever root canal takes place, a careful selection of material is important to prevent inflammatory reactions that may extend into the adjacent maxillary sinuses.

AIR POLLUTION

As part of the respiratory system, the nose and sinuses are designed to process air—to bring in oxygen that will be used by the cells to make energy, and to dispose of the waste product carbon dioxide. When you breathe in other substances along with oxygenated air, they are considered to be pollutants. Air pollution plays a significant role in sinus disease. Over the last few decades, there has been a major increase in urban air pollutants, and not coincidentally, a corresponding rise in the incidence of allergies, asthma, and sinusitis. Outdoors, smog permeated with ozone and other toxins acts as an irritant to

FACTORS IN POLLUTANT-INDUCED SINUSITIS

Various factors influence whether or not a pollutant will cause sinus disease. These include:

- The concentration and toxicity of the pollutant, and how long you are exposed to it.
- Whether or not other pollutants are present
- The status of your overall health, nutritional intake, and immune system
- Your respiratory rate
- Any preexisting sinus abnormalities or sinus or nasal disease
- Environmental factors such as temperature and humidity

delicate mucous membranes and may cause or aggravate infection. Indoor air is even worse—it has been identified by the EPA (Environmental Protection Agency) as one of the top five environmental health risks of our time.

Your Nasal Defenses

Healthy respiratory tracts can usually stand up well to pollutants. Your nose and sinuses typically act as efficient filters, routinely destroying millions of irritating particles, chemicals, and microorganisms in the air you breathe. The body's natural defensive responses include mucociliary clearance, reflexes, immune reactions, and antimicrobial action. For example, when you inhale a chemical vapor, you will probably find yourself sneezing as your body attempts to expel it. But your respiratory organs can do only so much, and as their defenses are gradually worn down by constant bombardment with pollutants, you become increasingly susceptible to infection. To further complicate matters, some of the body's own defensive responses—such as inflammation—also increase your vulnerability to sinusitis.

Outdoor Air Pollution

Outdoor air pollution is clearly associated with an aggravation of respiratory illnesses such as asthma, bronchitis, and sinusitis. Its most well-known manifestation is smog, which forms when moisture condenses on fine particles in the air. Smog—a term coined from the combination of "smoke" and "fog"—is a mixture of noxious gases and fine-particle pollutants. On hot summer days, it forms a toxic, yellowish brown haze over major urban areas.

Ozone

A major constituent of smog, ozone is generated by a complex photochemical reaction involving hydrocarbons, nitrogen oxides, and sunlight. Industrial emissions may travel for hundreds of miles on westerly winds until activated by the sun's powerful rays on hot summer days. Often cities will issue an alert when the concentration of ozone in the air grows dangerously elevated, recommending that the very young and the elderly remain indoors.

Ozone is an oxidant that can directly damage body tissues. It may lead to sinus inflammation, reduced mucociliary clearance, increased

SINUS AND NASAL RESPONSES TO INHALED POLLUTANTS

- The irritation response, which includes burning eyes and nose, tearing, coughing, headaches, and reflex holding of the breath.
- Inflammatory responses, such as widening of blood vessels (vasodilation), an abnormal accumulation of fluid in body tissues (edema), and an increase in leukocytes (white blood cells).
- Compromised immunity, as inhaled pollutants wear down your resistance and open the door to infection. Immunity can also be compromised by the direct toxic effects of pollutants. Mechanisms may include impaired mucociliary clearance.
- Impaired mucociliary clearance, meaning that mucus thickens and cilia become less effective in moving along the mucous blanket. This causes the retention of secretions and prolonged contact with pollutants, leading to a vicious cycle of further epithelial damage and immune dysfunction.
- Damage to the respiratory epithelium (the mucous membrane lining sinus and nasal passages), which increases its susceptibility to invasion by bacteria and other microorganisms.
- Increased nasal airflow resistance, especially in people who are sensitive to the effects of inhaled chemicals (such as those with multiple chemical sensitivity syndrome).

production of mucus, disturbances among mucous-producing cells, and possibly lowered immunity to infection. By irritating respiratory membranes, ozone can cause or worsen sinusitis. It is important to distinguish this ground-level pollutant from the protective layer of stratospheric ozone and is itself rapidly being depleted by pollutants such as car emissions.

Nitrogen Dioxide

Like ozone, nitrogen dioxide is a product of a photochemical reaction. It may be the result of either outdoor or indoor pollution. Nitrogen dioxide causes reduced mucociliary clearance and is associated with an increase in respiratory infections. Also like ozone, it is an oxidant and can cause direct tissue damage.

Sulfur Dioxide

Another important element of outdoor air pollution, sulfur dioxide is the result primarily of the burning of coal and fossil fuels. A small amount is also produced by volcanic eruptions. In contrast to ozone and nitrogen oxide, this is a water-soluble compound that is easily absorbed by nasal mucosa. High concentrations result in reduced mucociliary clearance. Sulfur dioxide can also convert to sulfuric acid, which is the chemical responsible for acid rain. In this form, it causes sinus problems including decreased mucociliary clearance and an increase of hyperreactivity in the airways.

Fine-Particle Pollutants

Fine particles suspended in the air can be due to either natural or synthetic sources. Natural sources include volcanic eruptions and soil erosion. But most commonly, fine-particle pollutants are the result of automobile exhaust, or the burning of coal, other fossil fuels, or wood. They include carbon and metal particles and metal oxides. Evidence indicates that fine-particle airborne pollutants make people more susceptible to upper respiratory infections.

Indoor Air Pollution

Studies conducted by the EPA have concluded that indoor air presents an even greater health hazard than outdoor air. Enclosed spaces are likely to contain a higher concentration of pollutants— and compounding the problem is the fact that most adults spend 90 percent of their time inside. In the home, the highest concentration of pollutants is typically in rooms where people smoke and in

---

HIDDEN HAZARDS AT THE OFFICE

- Pesticides sprayed by exterminators
- Printers, copiers, and fax machines that emit ozone
- Carbonless copy paper (the kind in credit card and bank receipts) that contains known carcinogens
- Renovations that generate paint fumes and dust
- Mold in walls
- Volatile organic chemicals (VOCs) that seep out of furniture, office equipment, and carpets
- Vents, located above parking lots, truck bays, or restaurants, that suck in harmful chemicals such as carbon monoxide
- Heating, ventilation, and air-conditioning (HVAC) systems that recirculate contaminated air
- Environmental tobacco smoke (ETS), or passive smoking

kitchens with gas stoves. Inside modern offices, workers are routinely exposed to pollutants that range from dizzying chemical fumes in new carpeting to solvents in paint that cause nose and sinus irritation. In commercial airplane cabins, ozone is typically present in a concentration three times higher than that permitted in outdoor air.

Sick Building Syndrome

In high-rise "sick buildings" built during the energy crisis of the 1970s, people can't even open a window to get a breath of fresh air. The insulation in these buildings is designed to retain heat—but in consequence, stagnant office air simply recirculates pollutants. You may have sick building syndrome (SBS) if you work in a sealed building and experience symptoms such as headaches, fatigue, dizziness, and difficulty concentrating. These symptoms ordinarily disappear when you leave the building. Associated with sick building syndrome is multiple chemical sensitivity (MCS). When you are affected with this syndrome, you become sensitive to nearly everything made with synthetic chemicals. Another problem is building-related illness (BRI), which is a more specific condition, with a readily identifiable cause in a particular building. Examples include Legionnaire's disease and building-related asthma.

THE SYMPTOMS OF SICK BUILDING SYNDROME

- Headache and eye, nose, or throat irritation
- Dizziness
- Nausea
- Fatigue
- Difficulty concentrating
- A heightened sensitivity to odors
- Cough
- Dry skin

Formaldehyde: A Ubiquitous Danger

Formaldehyde—an organic compound that is found virtually everywhere in our society—is a major indoor air hazard. It is an irritant to mucous membranes, reduces mucociliary clearance, and has been implicated in many cases of sick building syndrome. Construction materials such as plywood, paneling, particle board, and insulation are probably the largest source of formaldehyde. As a result, people who live in mobile homes are regularly exposed to very high levels of this cancer-causing pollutant. Unfortunately, due to its ubiquitous nature, it would be hard to completely rid one's environment of formaldehyde. However, you can take action to seal off formaldehyde-emitting surfaces. Alternatively, you can surround yourself to as great a degree as possible with natural products made without toxic chemicals. If you plan to install wall-to-wall carpeting or insulation in your home, closely question manufacturers or contractors about chemicals used in the materials you are thinking of buying.

FORMALDEHYDE-RELATED PRODUCTS

Even though the EPA declared formaldehyde to be a probable human carcinogen (cancer-causing agent) in 1987, an astonishing number of items still include this compound. Among them are:

Adhesives	Leather
Carpeting	Paints
Concrete	Paneling
Cosmetics	Paper
Deodorants	Particle board
Detergents	Pesticides
Dyes	Plastics
Explosives	Plywood
Fertilizers	Preservatives
Fiber board	Processed food
Foam insulation	Rubber
Fuels	Textiles
Furniture	Water softeners
Insulation	

Cigarette Smoke

Not surprisingly, children who are exposed to environmental tobacco smoke have more respiratory infections—including sinusitis—than those who enjoy smoke-free homes. Cigarette smoke contains thousands of chemicals, and dozens of these—such as the hydrocarbons benzene and tolulene—are known carcinogens. Of course, if you actually smoke cigarettes, you are exposing yourself to even more toxins and greater health risks overall than when you breathe in secondhand smoke. Heavy smoking causes nasal irritation and inflammation. Continuing to smoke when you have a sinus infection can make it worse. Gas pumps, automobile exhaust, dry cleaning, and room air fresheners are other sources of some of the same carcinogens and respiratory irritants found in cigarettes.

Gas Appliances

Gas stoves and other gas appliances emit nitric oxide, which rapidly oxidizes to nitrogen dioxide—a pollutant with effects such as tissue damage and the reduction of mucociliary clearance. In one study, children under the age of two who lived in homes with gas stoves experienced more frequent respiratory infections than children in homes that had electric stoves. Although nitrogen oxide is better known as a component of smog, only time will tell if it causes even more damage as an indoor air pollutant. If you have a gas stove, make sure your kitchen is well ventilated when you use it. Keep young children out of the kitchen when you are cooking, and if your child has respiratory problems, consider replacing gas appliances with electric ones.

LIMIT YOUR EXPOSURE TO POLLUTANTS

- Unless you suffer from seasonal allergies, open a window. Alternatively, install a ceiling fan.
- Remove all known pollutants from your home or office. For example, throw away any unused paint, solvents, or cleansers.
- Avoid using toxic chemical cleansers or pesticides. Choose natural products instead.
- Discontinue use of scented products such as room air fresheners.
- Air out dry-cleaned clothes before wearing them.
- Seal off formaldehyde-emitting surfaces. (See page 57 for a list of formaldehyde-related products.)
- Discontinue use of gas burners.
- When you are working around irritating fumes, protect your respiratory passages by wearing a mask.
- Install an air filter or purifier to clean home or office air. The best filters use a high efficiency particle accumulation (HEPA) system.
- Quit smoking, or at least smoke only outdoors.

BAROTRAUMA: SINUS DAMAGE DUE TO CHANGES IN AMBIENT PRESSURE

Activities such as air travel and scuba diving can also cause inflammation of the mucous membranes and problems with sinus drainage. Remember that your sinuses are small air-filled cavities connected to the nose and outside air by tiny openings called ostia. Consequently, they are easily affected by changes in outside air or water pressure. This is especially the case if you already have a cold or sinus infection, which pressure changes can worsen. Sinus damage related to changes in outside or ambient pressure is known as barotrauma.

SINUSITIS AND PRESSURE CHANGES

- In air travel, barotrauma is most likely to occur in small planes with unpressurized cabins or during military maneuvers where abrupt altitude and pressure changes are standard.
- If scuba divers fail to descend and ascend gradually, they can suffer severe injuries due to changes in water pressure.
- In the hospital, physicians are careful in their administration of hyperbaric oxygen therapy (increasing the oxygen supply in tissues by exposing a person to oxygen at a higher-than-normal atmospheric pressure), in order to prevent barotrauma.

IMMUNE PROBLEMS

Immune impairment is increasingly seen as a key element of chronic sinusitis. People who have immune problems are by definition more susceptible to infections of all kinds, including sinusitis. Of course, not everyone who suffers from chronic sinus disease is immunodeficient. But studies have shown that in many people who undergo repeated sinus surgery, an underlying immune defect is eventually uncovered. When sinusitis is related to immune impairment, there are more associated problems. An affected person may be less able to fight off even a simple infection; often more destructive and aggressive organisms are at work; and serious complications—such as the spread of infection into the orbits or brain—are more common.

Immune problems may be congenital or acquired. Some people are born with immune deficiencies—such as selective IgA (immunoglobulin A) deficiency (SIAD) or common variable immunodeficiency (CVID). Others have acquired immune problems. This group includes people who are taking corticosteroids for inflammatory conditions such as rheumatoid arthritis or ulcerative colitis, those who are undergoing radiation or chemotherapy for cancer, individuals who have had transplants and are taking powerful drugs to prevent their immune systems from rejecting the new organs, and people with HIV infection or AIDS.

HIV and AIDS

Sinusitis occurs in nearly seven out of ten people who are infected with HIV (the human immunodeficiency virus). Moreover, infection is usually more severe in HIV-positive individuals. It tends to affect multiple sinuses, to be more resistant to antibiotic therapy, and to involve infection with more obscure organisms. The development of sinus disease is usually associated with declining CD4+ lymphocyte counts. In HIV-infected children, sinusitis is the fourth most frequently reported infection (following ear infections, pneumonia, and skin and soft tissue infections). People with AIDS are also more vulnerable to a particularly virulent form of fungal sinusitis, known as acute or fulminant fungal sinusitis.

FUNGAL INFECTION

In recent years, scientists have focused increased attention on the role that fungi play in sinusitis. Fungi appear to be nearly ubiquitous in our environment. At the Mayo Clinic, in studies conducted by Dr. Jens Ponikau, these adaptable organisms were found in the sinuses of all normal subjects and in 96 percent of those with chronic sinusitis. There are several possible reasons for the increasing recognition of the role that fungi play in sinsusitis:

- Technical advances have led to improvements in the detection of fungal sinus disease.
- Widespread use of broad-spectrum antibiotics has led to fungal overgrowth in the nose and sinuses. Of particular concern is antibiotic use in plants and livestock, and our subsequent ingestion of the livestock. This may result in decreased immunity in otherwise healthy individuals.

- There are increasing numbers of people with immunosuppression, whether due to diseases such as diabetes mellitus or to decreased immunity following radiation, chemotherapy, transplants, or the chronic use of steroids.

What Are Fungi?

Fungi are simple but extremely adaptive organisms that are able to thrive in a variety of environments. They reproduce by simple division or spore formation. Throughout history, fungi have played a prominent role in the public health arena. For example, fungal contamination of the potato harvest was the source of the Great Famine in mid-nineteenth-century Ireland. In the twentieth century, the discovery of penicillin, which is derived from a mold, had a resounding impact on public health.

The Different Types of Fungal Sinus Disease

There are two primary types of fungal sinus disease: noninvasive and invasive. Because fungal disease attacks the nose as well as the sinuses, it is generally referred to as rhinosinusitis. Although the noninvasive form was virtually unknown until the last several years, today more and more doctors are coming to recognize this form of sinusitis. Each of the major forms of fungal sinus disease can be further broken down into subcategories:

Noninvasive Fungal Rhinosinusitis
- Superficial sinonasal mycosis
- Fungal ball
- Allergic fungal rhinosinusitis

Invasive Fungal Rhinosinusitis
- Chronic invasive fungal rhinosinusitis
- Acute (fulminant) fungal rhinosinusitis

Noninvasive Fungal Disease

This type of fungal rhinosinusitis is a reaction to fungi that are colonizers but not invaders of the sinuses. Noninvasive fungal sinus disease affects primarily individuals who do not have specific, active

---

SYMPTOMS OF FUNGAL SINUS DISEASE

- Nasal congestion and obstruction
- Blurred vision and other visual disturbances
- Facial pain
- Focal neurological deficits
- Headaches
- Olfactory disturbances, such as odors that other people do not smell
- Protrusion or bulging of the eyeball (proptosis)
- Seizures
- Sensorium disturbances (which affect consciousness and intellectual functions)

---

immune problems. Infection may be triggered by factors such as a genetic tendency toward allergies, especially immunoglobulins (Ig)E-mediated allergy.

Superficial Sinonasal Mycosis
This is the mildest form of fungal sinus disease. It occurs most often in people who have recently undergone sinus surgery and are consequently experiencing dry nasal passages or mucous retention. There may be no symptoms at all, or mild symptoms such as crusty debris when the nose is blown. Some people report detecting odors that others cannot smell.

Fungal Ball
This is a dense tangle of threadlike fungal parts called hyphae. A fungal ball may accompany cases of chronic or recurrent acute sinusitis, and is also seen with asthma. As with superficial sinonasal mycosis, sometimes there are no symptoms. In other cases, you may experience nasal congestion, obstruction, discharge, fever, cough, and blurred vision. Less commonly, there is facial pain, pressure, swelling, or headache. Fungal balls are more common in women than men.

Allergic Fungal Rhinosinusitis
Researchers disagree on the exact definition of allergic fungal sinusitis (AFS). Some consider it to be an allergy, others an infection, and still others say it is a combination of the two. AFS is a chronic condition with symptoms that range from mild to severe. In some cases, there are only mild allergic manifestations, polyps, and scattered fun-

gal hyphae. Others experience severe allergic symptoms, extensive fungal infection, and orbital and brain complications. AFS should be suspected in people who have a history of nasal polyps, prior sinus surgery, and asthma. It is characterized by the presence of both fungi and allergy-activated eosinophils.

Eosinophilia and Allergic Fungal Rhinosinusitis

Eosinophilia—an inflammatory tissue response—is increasingly regarded by researchers as an important factor in chronic sinusitis. Eosinophils—white blood cells that are commonly involved in allergic reactions—release destructive products such as major basic protein (MBP). Normally, eosinophils are important in the destruction of parasites, whereas neutrophils are important in the destruction of other bacteria.

Scientists at the Mayo Clinic have found that fungi are ubiquitous in the mucus that lines the sinuses. Thus fungi in immunologically competent people are not pathogens (disease-causing organisms). However, in some individuals there is a massive eosinophilic response causing the release of inflammatory mediators, which in turn leads to chronic sinusitis. Following the release of the mediators, bacteria can invade the sinus tissue.

Asthma and allergies are rare in indigenous populations where parasitic infections are common from shortly after birth onward. This has resulted in speculation that parasites play an important role in the evolution of immunological homeostasis (the constant internal environment that is required for bodily health). Eosinophils—one of whose basic functions is to destroy parasites—may have become misdirected in chronic sinusitis.

Invasive Fungal Rhinosinusitis

In this type of fungal sinus disease, there is an invasion of sinonasal tissue by fungal organisms. There are two types of invasive fungal rhinosinusitis: chronic invasive fungal rhinosinusitis and acute (fulminant) fungal rhinosinusitis. The chronic form is most common in people with competent immune systems. Acute fungal rhinosinusitis is a severe, life-threatening disease that attacks those with weakened immune systems (such as AIDS patients or those who have received bone marrow or organ transplants). When fungi invade tissue, it is essential to identify and control any underlying immune problem. Sometimes this is obvious, such as when a person is having radiation

CONDITIONS ASSOCIATED WITH INVASIVE FUNGAL INFECTIONS	
Acute leukemia	Immunologic disorders
Aplastic anemia	Lymphoma
Severe burns	Malnutrition
Chemotherapy and radiation	Multiple myeloma
Chronic use of corticosteroids	Renal failure
Diabetes mellitus	Organ transplantation
Gastroenteritis	

treatment or aggressive chemotherapy for cancer. Other times—such as when someone has undiagnosed diabetes—the issue is more subtle.

Chronic Invasive Fungal Rhinosinusitis

Also known as chronic indolent fungal sinusitis, this is a relatively rare but life-threatening disease. Chronic invasive fungal rhinosinusitis is characterized by headaches, nasal congestion, and other symptoms of chronic sinusitis. There may also be visual changes and protrusion or bulging of the eyeball (proptosis). This insidious disease progresses slowly, over a period of months to years. However, its slow-growing mass can eventually invade other structures—including the orbits and brain—and cause death. *Aspergillus* is the organism most commonly responsible for chronic invasive fungal rhinosinusitis.

Acute Fungal Rhinosinusitis

This rapidly progressive, often lethal disease occurs almost entirely in people with compromised immune systems. As the population of individuals with immune impairment has significantly risen (due to causes such as the increase in transplants and the widespread use of aggressive chemotherapy), acute fungal rhinosinusitis has also grown more common. If you have a known immune deficiency (for example, if you are taking a long course of corticosteroids) and experience sinusitis symptoms, your doctor should always check for dangerous fungal involvement. *Mucor* is the organism most commonly associated with acute fungal rhinosinusitis, although *Aspergillus* and other fungi are also sometimes involved. In the advanced stages of *Mucor* infection, the mucous membranes in the nose are covered with black scabs, or eschar. Unless the underlying cause of immunosuppression can be controlled, acute fungal rhinosinusitis is rapidly fatal.

MORE CAUSES OF SINUSITIS

In the last two chapters, we have covered many causes of sinus disease, from viral upper respiratory tract infections (the most common cause) to obscure genetic diseases that contribute to sinusitis and nasal polyps. But there are also a number of other less frequent causes. For example, sinusitis can be associated with systemic causes such as pregnancy, hypothyroidism, or Wegener's granulomatosis (a rare disorder characterized by areas of persistent tissue inflammation in the nasal passages, lungs, and kidneys). It can also develop as a side effect of certain medications, including birth control pills and antihypertensives such as beta-blockers. All these multiple factors make the differential diagnosis of sinus disease a special challenge to physicians.

CHAPTER 5

Making the Diagnosis

As is no doubt clear by now, sinusitis can be a baffling disease. Symptoms may be the result of infectious, noninfectious, or allergic syndromes, and often there is more than one underlying cause. Moreover, the symptoms of sinusitis mimic those of many other disorders. An acute case can easily be mistaken for a common cold, while chronic symptoms can be disturbing but subtle. In this chapter, we will help you sort through some confusing issues about diagnosis, such as when to consult your physician and how to locate the doctor who can best help you. You'll also learn what to expect as your doctor goes about determining the cause of your symptoms, from physical examination to the different types of tests he or she may order. Finally, diagnosis also includes testing for complications and underlying disorders.

WHEN TO CONSULT YOUR PHYSICIAN

In some cases of upper respiratory disease—such as when you have a common cold—it is not always necessary to see your doctor. But it's better to be safe than sorry. Keep in mind that if it is left untreated, chronic disease can cause permanent structural damage in the sinuses and lead to serious—possibly even life-threatening—complications. If you experience cold symptoms that last for longer than ten days, chances are that you have an acute sinus infection. See your doctor. If you experience vague symptoms—such as nasal congestion and discharge accompanied by headaches or fatigue—that linger for week after week, ask your doctor whether chronic sinusitis might be the problem. It is also essential to seek medical attention if your symptoms progress—for example, if you develop a fever, severe cough, facial pain, or ear or throat discomfort. In addition, physicians recommend that people who have an underlying immune condition (for example, decreased immunity because of taking steroids or undergoing chemotherapy, or due to a disease such as diabetes or HIV) always seek medical attention when they experience even more mild sinusitis symptoms. If you have other respiratory illnesses—such as asthma or emphysema—again you must see your doctor. A sinus infection can aggravate these problems. For example, if you have asthma, staying on top of sinusitis can mean that you do not have to take as many medications to control your condition.

CHOOSING THE RIGHT DOCTOR

Finding a physician who is trained in the diagnosis of sinusitis is an important first step in managing your disease. Unfortunately, in today's era of managed care, it often seems as if we don't have a lot of choices. For many people, a visit to the primary-care physician is mandatory before proceeding elsewhere. Correspondingly, children should see their regular pediatrician. The good news is that most primary-care practitioners can successfully diagnose and treat standard cases of acute sinus disease. On the other hand, if a diagnosis remains wanting or symptoms persist, don't be afraid to get a second opinion. And when two courses of antibiotics fail to control sinusitis, definitely ask for a referral to a specialist. Other indications for seeking a specialist's evaluation are recurrent or chronic sinusitis, a compromised immune system, and deteriorating condition. Any person with a complication always requires specialized care.

Depending upon your particular condition and needs, your primary-care practitioner may refer you to an otolaryngologist (a physician who has received advanced training in ear, nose, and throat disorders), an allergist (a specialist in diagnosing and treating allergies), or a pulmonologist (a specialist in lung disease) for further evaluation and treatment. An otolaryngologist—also known as an ENT, or ear, nose, and throat doctor—treats patients both medically and

surgically. If you have a sinus blockage, he or she can perform procedures such as draining infection and restoring normal mucociliary
clearance through the osteomeatal unit. An otolaryngologist is also
better qualified and has more experience in the treatment of complex
cases of sinusitis, such as those that involve an underlying fungal
infection or orbital or intracranial complications. If your sinus disease appears to be related to allergies, you may be referred to an allergist. This type of specialist can conduct tests to determine the triggers
of your allergies, and prescribe medication to control them. (Some
otolaryngologists also treat allergies.) A pulmonologist treats patients
in whom chronic sinus disease is linked with underlying lung disorders such as asthma.

WHEN TO SEE A SPECIALIST

In certain cases, your primary-care physician will refer you to a specialist such as an otolaryngologist. These circumstances include:

- If you suffer from recurrent or chronic sinusitis
- If your condition is deteriorating
- If your sinus disease fails to respond to two courses of antibiotic
  treatment
- If your immune system is somehow compromised (for example, if
  you have diabetes or HIV infection, or if you are undergoing radiation or chemotherapy)
- If you are hospitalized due to the severity of your infection or its
  complications

THE ELEMENTS OF DIAGNOSIS

Episodes of acute sinusitis are usually diagnosed on a clinical basis.
This means that your physician will thoroughly examine you, ask you
questions about your medical history, and on this basis make a deter-
mination as to whether or not you have sinus disease. In a simple,
uncomplicated case of acute sinusitis, usually no further action is necessary. Once the diagnosis is made, your doctor will send you home
with a prescription for antibiotics. Decongestants, mucous thinners,
and steroid nasal sprays may also be recommended. Of course, it's a
different story if you suffer from chronic symptoms (such as persis-

tent congestion, discharge, facial pain, coughing, or headache), if you experience recurrent episodes of acute sinusitis, or if sinusitis does not respond to medical therapy. In these kinds of cases, a more thorough workup is necessary, and your doctor may recommend other tests. But whatever type of sinusitis you have, chances are that your physician will begin by taking an in-depth medical history, which is a key element of diagnosis.

DIAGNOSING SINUS DISEASE

Diagnostic measures your physician takes may include the following:

- Medical history
- Physical examination
- Nasal endoscopy
- Imaging studies
- Laboratory studies

Taking a Medical History

Before conducting a physical examination, your doctor will take a thorough medical history. You can expect to be asked detailed questions about past episodes of sinusitis, and whether you also suffer from allergies or other health problems. In particular, your physician is apt to inquire into any personal or family history of lung diseases such as asthma or cystic fibrosis, or of immune disorders such as diabetes or aplastic anemia. Because environmental pollutants are believed to play an increasingly prominent role in sinus disease, your home and work environments may also be examined. If you smoke, it's important to tell your doctor, and you should let him or her know about all drugs you take.

The Physical Examination

A complete physical is the next step toward the diagnosis of sinusitis. Your physician will first check general health measures such as your height, weight, and blood pressure. Next he or she may listen to your lungs and examine your head and neck. In some cases, you may be asked to produce a sample of nasal discharge for analysis. As the doctor focuses more specifically on sinus-related phenomena, he or she

What are your symptoms? For example, are you experiencing nasal congestion or a purulent discharge? Do you have facial pain or pressure? What is the exact location of your pain? What about headaches, or ear, throat, or dental pain?

Is your pain better or worse when you keep your head upright? How about when you lie down, bend forward, cough, or strain?

Have you noticed any changes in your sense of smell or taste?

Are your eyes tired and swollen? Do they tear frequently?

Do you have a persistent cough? Is it productive or unproductive? When do you find yourself coughing most?

Are you unusually fatigued?

When did your symptoms begin?

Have you experienced these symptoms before?

Do symptoms appear worse at some times than others? For example, do they bother you more at night and early in the morning?

Do symptoms appear worse in certain locations (such as at your office or in the locker room at the gym)?

Do you have any history of sinus disease?

Have you recently had a cold or flu?

How often do you experience upper respiratory infections?

Do you have allergies or asthma? If you have allergies, what type? What triggers your reactions? Are your allergies worse at certain times of year?

Does anyone else in your family have a history of sinusitis or other respiratory diseases?

Are you pregnant?

Do you smoke?

Do people around you at home or at work smoke?

Do you have pets? If so, what type of pets and how long have you had them?

Have you recently made any changes in your life? Have you moved or changed jobs? Have you remodeled your home, or switched to a new perfume?

Do you eat nourishing foods and get enough sleep? Do you drink alcohol?

Have you recently been flying or scuba diving?

What type of heating and air-conditioning systems do you have in your home?

What over-the-counter and prescription medications do you take? Are you taking medications such as birth control pills or antihypertensives, which can cause congestion?

Are you allergic to any medications? Are you sensitive to aspirin?

will be on the lookout for a number of characteristic physical findings of sinus disease, such as a thickened nasal discharge and swelling of the mucous membranes inside your nose. To that end, your nose, throat, and ears will be visually examined with the aid of a nasal speculum and a mirror that reflects light from a light source up into the nose. This examination is generally not painful or even uncomfortable. Other observations that contribute to a diagnosis of sinusitis include nasal polyps, inflammation of the turbinates, tenderness when the skin over the infected sinuses is touched, and swollen eyelids. If eye complications are suspected, examination should include an assessment of visual acuity. The loss of perception of the color red is an early sign of a problem. Your doctor will also look for decreased mobility of the eye and any bulging of the eyeball. Whenever the diagnosis of sinusitis is in doubt—or if your doctor believes that the infection is widespread, or there are complications—further testing is necessary.

PHYSICAL FINDINGS IN SINUSITIS

Thickened, purulent nasal discharge
Swelling, redness, and congestion of the nasal mucosa
Chronic mild throat inflammation
Tenderness over infected sinuses
Swollen eyelids
Tearing
Nasal polyps
Inflammation and swelling of the middle and inferior turbinates in the nose
A retracted eardrum

DIAGNOSTIC TESTS

Although clinical evaluation can be sufficient in and of itself in the diagnosis of acute sinusitis, chronic or recurrent cases often require further testing. Diagnostic nasal endoscopy is usually the first test your doctor will recommend. An endoscope is a viewing device with a lens mounted on a long tube. It allows your doctor to look directly inside the accessible areas of your sinuses and obtain a nasal culture. Although laboratory studies are unnecessary in acute flare-ups, cultures can identify the responsible infective organisms in stubborn chronic or recurrent cases.

Imaging or radiologic studies are normally the next step. By using these techniques, your doctor can examine the inside of your sinuses and surrounding structures without invasive tests or surgery. X rays, CT (computerized tomography) scanning, and MRI (magnetic resonance imaging) display nasal and sinus anatomy, and to a greater or lesser extent reveal the nature and exact location of osteomeatal obstruction. Physicians agree that cross-sectional imaging modalities (such as CT and MRI) are far superior to plain films (that is, X rays). By taking many cross-sectional pictures from a number of different angles, and then combining them, these devices provide more accurate and complete imaging of the sinuses. Of the three modalities commonly used for evaluating sinusitis, CT scanning is the most effective and X rays the least.

ABOUT LABORATORY STUDIES

- Laboratory studies are usually *not* necessary in the diagnosis of acute sinus disease. They play a greater role in the diagnosis of chronic or recurrent sinusitis, and may aid in the detection of underlying illnesses.
- In children who experience recurrent acute sinusitis or nasal polyps, physicians often recommend the following laboratory studies:

    A sweat chloride test for cystic fibrosis
    Allergy tests

Nasal Endoscopy

Nasal endoscopy is one of the greatest advances in the diagnosis of sinusitis in recent years. This is ordinarily the first test performed by your physician and should precede any imaging study. Endoscopy is performed with the aid of a rigid, rodlike, fiberoptic instrument that the doctor uses to look inside the drainage passageways from the sinuses. An endoscope is basically a long, narrow tube—it is about 3 to 4 millimeters in diameter, and never penetrates more than 7 to 8 centimeters into the nose. Before endoscopy, you will be given a local anesthetic and decongestant to lessen any discomfort. The procedure takes only minutes.

Endoscopy is used to examine the middle meatus and assess the osteomeatal unit (OMU), which is the seat of sinus disease. If the procedure reveals symptoms such as blockage of the osteomeatal unit, your doctor will make a diagnosis of sinus disease. Endoscopy is also sometimes used to remove a sample of mucus to culture in the laboratory. The nasal cultures from this procedure are more like those obtained by surgical aspiration than by a simple nasal swab, so they can give your doctor a more accurate idea of what is going on in your sinuses. The culture is sent to the laboratory to see what type of organism it grows. This will help your doctor decide on the best type of antibiotic or other (for example, antifungal) medication for your particular case of sinusitis. (See also chapter 7, in which we discuss functional endoscopic sinus surgery, or FESS.)

X Rays

Also known as plain films or radiographs, X rays are still the most frequently used imaging tests in the diagnosis of sinusitis. Unfortunately, they are far from the most accurate, as plain films fail to show the extent of disease. X rays are helpful on a limited basis. For instance, those known as the Caldwell's and Water's views successfully display the air and fluid levels in the maxillary and frontal sinuses. However, X rays are the least accurate modality for displaying disease in the more remote ethmoids and elsewhere around the sinuses and their surrounding structures. Studies have also shown that there is a high rate of false-positive results from standard radiographs. This means that some people are diagnosed with sinusitis, and perhaps needlessly treated, when they don't even have the disease. X rays are generally much less accurate than CT scans, which are the gold standard of imaging studies for sinus disease.

ABOUT IMAGING STUDIES

- Although they are still commonly used, plain X rays are the least accurate imaging modality for the evaluation of sinus disease.
- Coronal CT scans are the gold standard of sinusitis diagnosis.
- MRI scans have two weaknesses:
    They do not display fine bony details.
    They are oversensitive in the detection of relatively insignificant details.

CT Scanning

The gold standard of imaging studies for this disease, CT scanning provides a clear display of the sinuses not afforded by any other imaging technique. Three types of CT—coronal, axial, and sometimes sagittal—are used to provide exquisitely detailed representations of the sinuses and their surrounding structures. Coronal CT scans are best, especially where endoscopic surgery is concerned. Their lucid representation of the bony detail of the osteomeatal unit and the nasal and sinus passages makes it possible for an otolaryngologist to see the relationship between a person's anatomy and his or her sinus disease, facilitating an accurate diagnosis and effective treatment. CT is particularly effective in detecting bony abnormalities that contribute to sinus disease but can be surgically corrected. CT findings that suggest a diagnosis of chronic sinusitis include: thickening of the mucous membranes, bony remodeling, multiple polyps (polyposis), bony thickening (due to osteitis), and osteomeatal obstruction.

CT is *not* recommended in the evaluation of simple, uncomplicated cases of acute sinusitis. In fact, in most cases it cannot distinguish between sinus abnormalities due to viral rhinitis (a common cold) and sinus abnormalities caused by acute bacterial sinusitis. However, this important diagnostic tool has a significant role in chronic and recurrent sinusitis and is especially beneficial in those who have complications or for whom surgery is being considered. In functional endoscopic sinus surgery (FESS), CT provides an invaluable "road map" for the surgeon to follow around a person's osteomeatal channels and other critical sinus structures. If three to four weeks of antibiotics fail to control sinusitis, CT is also recommended. It is superior in its display of sinus anatomy, including possible abnormalities. CT also plays a critical role in tracking the extent of disease and patient outcome.

HAVING A CT SCAN

Computerized tomography (CT) scanning is the imaging technique of choice for sinusitis. This method displays detailed images of the sinuses, nasal passages, and related structures such as the orbits. During the procedure, you lie on a motorized bed and are moved into a scanner. In order to prevent blurring of images, you will be asked to stay completely still while the images are taken. The procedure takes about thirty minutes. If you are anxious, ask your doctor to give you a sedative beforehand.

MRI

Magnetic resonance imaging uses radio waves, a powerful magnet, and a computer to create cross-sectional images. Today this procedure is more readily available and also less expensive than it was in the past. MRI has certain disadvantages in the diagnosis of sinus disease. Notably, unlike CT, this technique cannot show fine bony details. It is unable to display the delicate bony anatomy of the sinuses and the intricate relationships among the various drainage structures. In addition, MRI overdiagnoses mucosal thickening, which can—and does—lead to the overdiagnosis of sinus disease. In the normal nasal cycle, there is a periodic congestion and decongestion of each side of the nasal turbinates, nasal septum, and ethmoid air cell mucosa. This takes place over a fifty-minute to six-hour period. Consequently, radiologists who are unaware of the nasal cycle mistake normal mucosal swelling of the nasal cycle for ethmoid sinusitis. But as you will see below, this is not to say that MRI doesn't have a valuable role in diagnosing the complications of sinusitis.

HAVING AN MRI

During an MRI, you are placed inside a tunnel in a large, powerful magnet. You must lie very still for up to an hour, as radio waves are passed through your body. Although there is no actual physical discomfort, some people find the experience claustrophobic. If you feel anxious, ask your physician for a sedative beforehand.

DIAGNOSING EYE AND BRAIN COMPLICATIONS

If your doctor suspects that you have orbital (eye) or intracranial (brain) complications, you will need to be admitted to a hospital for further evaluation. There you will be examined by specialists such as an otolaryngologist, an ophthalmologist (a specialist in eye disorders), a neurologist (a physician who is specially trained in diseases of the brain and nervous system), and/or a neurosurgeon (a specialist trained in surgery of the brain and nervous system).

The primary imaging techniques used to diagnose serious complications are CT scanning and MRI. In addition to detecting complications, these tests can distinguish their relative severity and monitor your response to treatment. They have gradually come to replace past tests such as carotid angiograms and radionuclide brain scans. CT is better at detecting the bony implications of complications such as orbital cellulitis and mucoceles, while MRI is adept at assessing their inflammation and involvement with other structures. MRI is particularly accurate in its depiction of soft tissue and inflammation and is considered superior to CT in the diagnosis of meningitis. MRI is also recommended in the evaluation of potential brain complications and in distinguishing between inflammatory and cancerous problems.

Other tests used in the diagnosis of complications include X rays and lumbar punctures. Although they are far from the most accurate modality, traditional X rays are still frequently ordered. A lumbar puncture (see below) is performed primarily when meningitis is suspected. Otherwise, its risks generally outweigh its benefits. This procedure is never performed without a previous CT scan to rule out mass effect that could lead to brain herniation at the time of puncture.

HAVING A LUMBAR PUNCTURE

A lumbar puncture is performed to search for evidence of meningitis. In this procedure, which takes place under local anesthesia, a health care professional inserts a hollow needle between two vertebrae near the base of your spine. The pressure of cerebrospinal fluid (the fluid that flows through your brain and spinal cord) is checked, and a sample is removed for analysis. The procedure takes about fifteen minutes. Afterward, in order to prevent a severe headache, you must remain lying down for an hour.

SPECIAL TESTS FOR UNDERLYING CONDITIONS

Because other conditions so often underlie and contribute to sinusitis, your doctor will also look for other diseases. Here we discuss the diagnosis of several disorders that are frequently linked with sinusitis.

Allergies

As with some cases of sinusitis, a detailed medical history and physical examination are sometimes all that is necessary to diagnose your allergies. Other times further testing is required. In these circumstances, you may be sent to a board-certified allergist or otolaryngologist for additional evaluation. Common tests they may perform include prick or patch tests, in which your skin is exposed to small amounts of allergens. If you are allergic to that substance, the skin around the area will redden and a small welt will form. This means that the IgE antibodies specific to the allergen have responded by triggering the release of histamine. An alternative to skin testing is a blood test known as RAST (Radioallergosorbent Test), which measures the level of allergen-specific IgE antibodies in the blood.

Asthma

An accurate diagnosis of asthma requires an objective measurement of lung function. If your physician suspects that you may have asthma, he or she will conduct assessments of breathing called spirometry, or pulmonary function tests. These measure the level of airflow obstruction in the lungs. Often spirometry can be performed right in your doctor's office. Other tests your doctor may order include imaging studies such as chest X rays, a complete blood count (CBC), allergy tests, bronchial provocation testing (to test your sensitivity to suspected triggers), or an exercise challenge (when exercise is a suspected trigger of symptoms).

Cystic Fibrosis

Cystic fibrosis is commonly diagnosed through a sweat test. This disease stimulates certain glands to produce abnormal amounts of salt, which are released through the body's sweat. In the test, a child's forearm is wrapped with a pad of gauze or filter paper to collect the sweat. A harmless chemical, along with a small amount of electricity, stimulates nearby glands to produce sweat. This is sent to the laboratory for analysis. If the test is positive, it is usually repeated.

Gastroesophageal Reflux

Diagnosis of gastroesophageal reflux can be made by medical history, through an esophagram (also known as a barium swallow or upper gastrointestinal [GI] series), and gastroscopy (visual examination of the esophagus, stomach, and duodenum using a slim, lighted tube called a gastroscope). The definitive test uses two tubes that measure acidity. One tube is placed in the distal esophagus and one tube is placed just above the esophagus. Measuring the pressure at different key points within the esophagus can also be helpful.

THE NEXT STEP: PROPER TREATMENT

Once your physician has obtained your medical history, examined you, and possibly performed tests to make an accurate diagnosis, the next step is to get proper treatment. In the following chapter, we discuss the medical treatment of sinus disease, and in chapter 7, we explain what you can expect when surgery is necessary.

CHAPTER 6

Medications for Sinusitis

Treatment with medications plays a crucial part in the management of sinusitis. The decision about which medicines are right for you depends upon the type of sinusitis you suffer from, as well as its underlying cause. Most commonly, antibiotics are prescribed to cure bacterial infections, while drugs like decongestants allow you to breathe better, and mucous thinners permit you to drain better. When inflammatory and immune factors come into play—as in chronic sinusitis—steroids are another important element of treatment. Doctors also prescribe medications for the complications of sinusitis, and for the treatment of related conditions. Ultimately, however, the success or failure of any medication depends in large part on the degree of responsibility that you are willing to assume for your own health and well-being.

TAKING RESPONSIBILITY

Making sure that you understand all aspects of your medical treatment is both your right and your responsibility. Once your doctor has written a prescription, it is up to you to follow through and take your medication correctly. A few basic guidelines can help you use sinusitis drugs safely and wisely:

• Follow your physician's instructions exactly: Do not skip doses, even if you feel better, and never change your medication program without consulting your doctor.

• Tell your physician if you have had an adverse reaction to this or any other related drug in the past.

• Make sure that your doctor knows of all other drugs you take, both prescription and over-the-counter. In addition, inform him or her about any alternative remedies and vitamin or mineral supplements that you use. For your own safety, it is also important to let your physician know if you drink alcohol or take illicit drugs.

• Tell your doctor about any other conditions you have, such as liver disease, high blood pressure, or diabetes.

• Always inform your doctor if you are pregnant or breast-feeding, or thinking about becoming pregnant. Drugs can negatively affect a growing baby or developing fetus.

• Contact your doctor at once if you develop any uncomfortable side effects.

• Don't hesitate to inquire further about any drugs your doctor recommends or prescribes.

ASK QUESTIONS

Never be afraid to ask questions about the drugs you take, especially when your doctor prescribes a new medication. A good working relationship is a key part of the effective management of sinusitis and related conditions. It may even be beneficial if your doctor's office can put your medication regimen in writing, for easy access by yourself and those close to you. In many cases, your pharmacist can also help you out. Pharmacies today computerize records and thus can quickly and easily tell you about any dangerous side effects or drug interactions. Ask these important questions before taking any new medication:

What are the generic and brand names of the medication I am taking?
Why is this medication prescribed?
How does this drug work in my body?
How long must I take it before my symptoms are relieved?
Should I continue taking this medication even if I no longer experience symptoms?

What should I do if medication does not relieve my symptoms?

How often should I take this drug?

What is the correct dosage?

If the drug is for a child, are there any special dosage considerations? Or other concerns?

Are there any special recommendations for seniors?

What if I have a preexisting condition, such as kidney or liver disease?

Is it preferable to take this medication at a certain time of day?

Should this drug be taken with food or on an empty stomach?

What should I do if I accidentally skip a dose?

What should I do if I accidentally take an extra dose?

Will this drug interact with any other prescription or over-the-counter medications that I take?

Can I take this medication along with vitamin and mineral supplements or alternative remedies?

What side effects should I expect?

Does this drug have any potentially dangerous adverse effects? What are their warning signs?

Will this medication affect other aspects of my life, such as my ability to participate in sports or exercise? Drive a car or concentrate at work? Sleep? Are there any special dietary concerns?

What should I do if I develop side effects or adverse reactions?

Where should I store this drug? For example, does it need to be refrigerated?

ACUTE SINUSITIS

Although undoubtedly less complicated than chronic disease, acute sinusitis poses its own set of problems and can be challenging to treat. Moreover, it is essential to cure acute disease before it spirals out of control and develops into a chronic or recurrent problem. Acute sinusitis usually develops as a result of an upper respiratory infection. Medications your doctor may recommend to control the infection and ease your symptoms include antibiotics, decongestants, mucous thinners, steroid nasal sprays, saline sprays, and anticholinergic nasal sprays. Unless there is an underlying allergic problem, antihistamines are not recommended.

Antibiotics

Antibiotics are the standard treatment for simple, uncomplicated acute sinus disease. Their goal is to restore the sinuses to health and to prevent the development of chronic sinus disease and brain or eye complications. Types of antibiotics prescribed for both acute and chronic sinusitis include the penicillin, cephalosporin, macrolide, sulfa, and fluoroquinolone groups. For acute disease, taking the medicine is recommended for a minimum of ten to fourteen days. Most people respond very well to this treatment, and few have resistant infections that develop into chronic or recurrent problems. But if symptoms continue after one course of antibiotics, your doctor will most likely prescribe an additional two weeks.

Which Antibiotic Is Right for You?

The choice of an appropriate antibiotic depends on the underlying organism responsible for your infection. Other considerations your doctor will take into account include your overall health, whether or not you are allergic to certain medications, possible side effects, and the length of time you must take the drug. Cost and convenience also come into play. For example, some newly approved antibiotics need be taken only once rather than several times a day. However, since there are no generic versions yet available, these are likely to be more expensive than older drugs. If your insurance plan does not cover medications or if cost is otherwise a concern, ask your doctor whether the older drug would be equally (or nearly equally) effective.

Are Nasal Cultures Necessary for Acute Sinusitis?

In chronic or recurrent cases of sinusitis, doctors usually take a nasal culture and analyze it to identify the responsible bacteria or other organism (such as fungi). This helps determine what antibiotic (or other medication) will be most effective against it. In most cases of simple, uncomplicated acute disease, no cultures are taken. But as the number of antibiotic-resistant bacteria rises, more and more doctors are choosing culture-directed antibiotics even for acute sinusitis. Nasal cultures are also recommended for anyone with immune impairment or in whom resistant infection is suspected.

Antibiotic-Resistant Bacteria on the Rise

Bacteria belong to a family of single-cell organisms that—unlike viruses and fungi—respond well to antibiotic treatment. But in recent years, there has been growing concern about the role that antibiotic-resistant organisms increasingly play in acute as well as chronic sinus disease. As you learned in chapter 1 (see page 6), the overuse of antibiotics has led to a new generation of supergerms—tough bacteria that stubbornly resist treatment with the use of traditional antibiotics. Reasons for this alarming new trend include the incorrect prescription of antibiotics for viruses (against which they do no good whatsoever), the habit of some people to stop taking antibiotics for bacterial infections once they feel well (which leads to the creation of more virulent, drug-resistant organisms), the wholesale feeding of antibiotics to chickens and other livestock (which then pass on increasingly drug-resistant bacteria to humans through the food chain), and the use of preventive (prophylactic) or long-term antibiotic regimens for infection. But whatever the underlying cause or causes may be, growing antibiotic resistance poses an enormous and increasing challenge to doctors. For example, amoxicillin was once the drug of choice for acute sinusitis—but as resistant bacteria have seized center stage, the newer, tougher, less bacteria-resistant antibiotics are more frequently and necessarily prescribed, instead of being reserved for more serious bacterial diseases.

Treatment For Mild Infections

Doctors make a distinction between mild and moderate cases of acute sinusitis. Mild infections are those that last for up to ten days, with symptoms such as a persistent runny nose and fatigue. The first group of antibiotics listed below is the one preferred for the treatment of mild disease. The effectiveness of the second group is limited, with a possible failure rate of 20 to 25 percent. In addition, Bactrim and related drugs have been associated with severe reactions such as toxic epidural necrolysis (also known as Stevens-Johnson syndrome, a life-threatening condition in which the skin blisters and peels off).

In adults with mild disease who have not taken antibiotics in the previous four to six weeks, doctors recommend primarily four drugs: amoxicillin (Amoxil and Trimox), amoxicillin-clavulanate (Augmentin), cefpodoxime proxetil (Vantin), and cefuroxime axetil (Ceftin). As you can see, most prescription drugs are known by two or more names: their chemical, or generic, name and the manufacturers' brand names. Following are descriptions of these four antibiotics:

Generic Name: Amoxicillin
Brand Names: Amoxil and Trimox
Amoxicillin is a penicillin antibiotic that kills bacteria by destroying their cell walls. Before taking this drug, inform your doctor if you are allergic to penicillin or to cephalosporin antibiotics. If so, you may also be allergic to amoxicillin, and your doctor will probably prescribe an alternate antibiotic.

Caution:
If your doctor prescribes this drug and you experience allergic symptoms (such as a skin rash, itching, swelling, fever, chills, muscle aches, breathing difficulties, or a sudden drop in blood pressure), stop taking amoxicillin at once and seek immediate medical attention.

Possible Side Effects:
Abdominal pain, upset stomach, nausea, vomiting, diarrhea, colitis, skin rash, itching, peeling skin, agitation, hyperactivity, confusion, changes in behavior, insomnia, liver problems, and anemia.

Possible Drug Interactions:
Check with your doctor before combining amoxicillin with other drugs. Chloramphenicol (Chloromycetin), erythromycin (E.E.S., E-Mycin, ERYC), and tetracycline (Achromycin or Sumycin) can decrease the effectiveness of amoxicillin. Probenecid (Benemid) can increase the blood level of amoxicillin.

Who Should Not Take This Drug:
Always tell your doctor if you are or think you may be pregnant, or if you are breast-feeding; only he or she can determine if it is safe for you to take this drug. Also inform your doctor if you have colitis, diabetes, or kidney or liver disease. This medication should not be taken if you have experienced a previous allergic reaction to penicillin or to a cephalosporin antibiotic.

How to Take This Drug:
Amoxicillin can be taken with or without food. However, to prevent stomach upset, it is best to take this drug with meals or snacks.

What to Do If You Miss a Dose:
Take it as soon as you remember. If it is almost time for the next dose, take the one you missed, and take the remaining doses at even inter-

vals throughout the rest of the day. Then return to your regular schedule.

Generic Name: Amoxicillin-clavulanate
Brand Name: Augmentin

Augmentin is a combination of amoxicillin and clavulanic acid—the clavulanic acid is said to "augment" the effectiveness of amoxicillin. Before taking this drug, inform your doctor if you are allergic to penicillin or to cephalosporin antibiotics. If so, you may also be allergic to Augmentin, and your doctor will most likely prescribe a different antibiotic.

Caution:

If your doctor prescribes this drug and you experience allergic symptoms (such as a skin rash, itching, swelling, fever, chills, muscle aches, breathing difficulties, or a sudden drop in blood pressure), stop taking Augmentin at once and seek immediate medical attention.

Possible Side Effects:

Abdominal pain, upset stomach, nausea, vomiting, diarrhea, gas, colitis, skin rash, hives, itching, peeling skin, itching or burning of the vagina, yeast infections, mouth sores, joint pain, muscle pain, headache, anemia, agitation, hyperactivity, confusion, changes in behavior, insomnia, liver and kidney problems.

Possible Drug Interactions:

Consult your doctor before combining Augmentin with other drugs. Chloramphenicol (Chloromycetin), erythromycin (E.E.S., E-Mycin, ERYC), and tetracycline (Achromycin or Sumycin) can decrease the effectiveness of Augmentin. Probenecid (Benemid) can increase the blood level of Augmentin. This drug may reduce the effectiveness of oral contraceptives.

Who Should Not Take This Drug:

Always tell your doctor about any medical conditions that you have, especially colitis, diabetes, or kidney or liver disease. This drug should not be taken if you have experienced a previous allergic reaction to penicillin or to a cephalosporin antibiotic. Also tell your doctor if you are or think you may be pregnant, or if you are breast-feeding; only he or she can determine if it is safe for you to take Augmentin.

How to Take This Drug:
Augmentin should always be taken with food.

What to Do If You Miss a Dose:
Take it as soon as you remember. If it is almost time for the next dose, take the one you missed, and take the remaining doses at even intervals throughout the rest of the day. Then return to your regular schedule.

Generic Name: Cefpodoxime proxetil
Brand Name: Vantin
Vantin is a cephalosporin antibiotic. The cephalosporins are similar to penicillin, and some people who are allergic to penicillin are also allergic to cephalosporins. Accordingly, always inform your doctor if you are allergic to any other cephalosporin antibiotic or to penicillin. If so, your doctor will probably prescribe a different antibiotic.

Caution:
If your doctor prescribes this drug and you experience allergic symptoms (such as breathing difficulties, a pounding heartbeat, a skin rash, or hives), stop taking Vantin at once and seek immediate medical attention.

Possible Side Effects:
Abdominal pain, upset stomach, nausea, vomiting, diarrhea, gas, colitis, skin rash, hives, itching, joint pain, muscle pain, chest tightness, headache, weakness, tiredness, tingling in the hands or feet, anemia, confusion, dizziness, appetite loss, altered sense of taste, changes in blood cells, and liver or kidney problems.

Possible Drug Interactions:
Check with your doctor before combining Vantin with other drugs. Vantin may interact with: antacids, loop diuretics, cimetidine (Tagamet), famotidine (Pepcid), ranitidine (Zantac), nizatidine (Axid), and probenecid (Benemid).

Who Should Not Take This Drug:
Always tell your doctor if you are or think you may be pregnant, or if you are breast-feeding; only he or she can determine whether it is safe for you to take this drug. Also inform your physician about any other

medical conditions that you have. Vantin should be used with caution (if at all) if you have kidney or liver disease. This drug should not be taken if you have experienced a previous allergic reaction to another cephalosporin antibiotic or to penicillin.

How to Take This Drug:
Vantin should always be taken with food.

What to Do If You Miss a Dose:
Take it as soon as you remember. If it is almost time for the next dose, take the one you missed, and take the remaining doses at even intervals throughout the rest of the day. Then return to your regular schedule.

Generic Name: Cefuroxime axetil
Brand Name: Ceftin
Like Vantin, Ceftin is a cephalosporin antibiotic. The cephalosporins are similar to penicillin, and some people who are allergic to penicillin are also allergic to cephalosporins. Tell your doctor if you are allergic to any other cephalosporin antibiotic or to penicillin, so he or she can prescribe a different antibiotic.

Caution:
If your doctor prescribes this drug and you experience allergic symptoms (such as breathing difficulties, a pounding heartbeat, a skin rash, or hives), stop taking Ceftin at once and seek immediate medical attention.

Possible Side Effects:
Nausea, vomiting, diarrhea, diaper rash in infants, abdominal pain, gas, indigestion, skin rash, hives, itching, appetite loss, mouth sores, joint pain, chest pain, headache, appetite loss, thirst, urinary problems, sleepiness, vaginitis, changes in blood cells, liver and kidney problems, and seizures.

Possible Drug Interactions:
Consult your doctor before taking Ceftin along with other drugs. This medication may interact with: antacids, loop diuretics, cimetidine (Tagamet), famotidine (Pepcid), ranitidine (Zantac), nizatidine (Axid), and probenecid (Benemid).

Who Should Not Take This Drug:

Always tell your doctor about any medical conditions that you have. Ceftin should be used with caution (if at all) if you have kidney disease. This medication should not be taken if you have experienced a previous allergic reaction to another cephalosporin antibiotic or to penicillin. Also inform your doctor if you are or think you may be pregnant, or if you are breast-feeding; only he or she can determine if it is safe for you to take this medication.

How to Take This Drug:

To prevent stomach upset, Ceftin tablets can be taken with milk or food. The oral suspension must be taken with food. Food increases the absorption of Ceftin.

What to Do If You Miss a Dose:

Take it as soon as you remember. If it is almost time for the next dose, take the one you missed, and take the remaining doses at even intervals throughout the rest of the day. Then return to your regular schedule.

Other Antibiotics for Mild Infections

If you are allergic to penicillin or cephalosporin drugs, such as those listed above, doctors recommend azithromycin (Zithromax), clarithromycin (Biaxin), doxycycline (Doryx), erythromycin (E.E.S., E-Mycin, and others), or trimethoprim-sulfamethoxazole (for example, Bactrim, Cotrim, and Septra). Following are descriptions of these medications:

Generic Name: Azithromycin
Brand Name: Zithromax

Zithromax is a macrolide antibiotic related to erythromycin. Before taking this drug, inform your doctor if you are allergic to erythromycin, or if you have experienced allergic reactions to similar antibiotics such as Biaxin. If so, you are probably allergic to Zithromax as well, and your doctor will prescribe a different antibiotic.

Caution:

If your doctor prescribes this drug and you experience allergic symptoms such as angiodema (severe swelling of the face, neck, and lips that interferes with speaking, swallowing, and breathing) or anaphylaxis (a life-threatening condition characterized by difficulty breathing, a rapid drop in blood pressure, rapid pulse, and paleness), stop taking Zithromax at once and seek immediate medical attention.

Possible Side Effects:
Abdominal pain, diarrhea, loose stools, gas, bloody stools, vomiting, indigestion, colitis, dizziness, headache, light sensitivity, heart palpitations, rash, vaginitis, yeast infections, kidney and liver problems.

Possible Drug Interactions:
Check with your doctor before combining Zithromax with other drugs. Zithromax may interact with: antacids that contain aluminum or magnesium (such as Gelusil or Maalox), carbamazepine (Tegretol), cyclosporine (Neoral and Sandimmune), digoxin (Lanoxin), lovastatin (Mevacor), phenytoin (Dilantin), triazolam (Halcion), warfarin (Coumadin), ergot-containing drugs, some antihistamines, and theophylline drugs.

Who Should Not Take This Drug:
Inform your doctor if you are or think you may be pregnant, or if you are breast-feeding; only he or she can determine if it is safe for you to take Zithromax. Also tell your doctor if you have liver disease. This drug should not be taken if you have experienced a previous allergic reaction to erythromycin.

How to Take This Drug:
Unlike other antibiotics, Zithromax is usually taken once a day for five days. Take the capsules and oral suspension one hour before or two hours after meals. The tablets can be taken with or without food. Do not take any form of Zithromax with antacids that contain aluminum or magnesium.

What to Do If You Miss a Dose:
Take it as soon as you remember. Do not try to catch up by doubling doses.

Generic Name: Clarithromycin
Brand Name: Biaxin
Like Zithromax, Biaxin is a macrolide antibiotic related to erythromycin. Before taking this drug, inform your doctor if you are allergic to erythromycin, or if you have experienced allergic reactions to similar antibiotics such as Zithromax. If so, you are probably

allergic to Biaxin as well, and your doctor will prescribe a different antibiotic.

Possible Side Effects:
Abdominal pain, diarrhea, nausea, vomiting, indigestion, rash, alterations in smell or taste, headache, behavior changes, dizziness, nightmares, insomnia, colitis, and liver problems.

Possible Drug Interactions:
Consult your doctor before taking Biaxin in conjunction with other drugs. This medication may interact with: bromocriptine (Parlodel), carbamazepine (Tegretol), cisapride (Propulsid), cyclosporine (Neoral and Sandimmune), disopyramide (Norpace), fluconazole (Diflucan), hexobarbital, lovastatin (Mevacor), phenytoin (Dilantin), pimozide (Orap), rifabutin (Mycobutin), ritonavir (Norvir), tacrolimus (Prograf), valproate (Depakene and Depakote), zidovudine (Retrovir), and theophylline drugs.

Who Should Not Take This Drug:
Always tell your doctor about any medical conditions that you have. This drug should not be taken if you have experienced a previous allergic reaction to erythromycin. Inform your doctor if you are or think you may be pregnant, or if you are breast-feeding; only he or she can determine if it is safe for you to take Biaxin.

How to Take This Drug:
Take regular Biaxin tablets and oral suspension with or without food. Take Biaxin XL with food.

What to Do If You Miss a Dose:
Take it as soon as you remember. If it is almost time for the next dose, take the one you missed, and take the remaining doses at even intervals throughout the rest of the day. Then return to your regular schedule.

Generic Name: Doxycycline
Brand Name: Doryx
Doryx is a broad-spectrum tetracycline antibiotic. Before taking Doryx, inform your doctor if you have ever experienced an allergic reaction to this or similar drugs, so he or she can prescribe a different antibiotic.

Caution:
If your doctor prescribes this drug and you experience allergic symptoms such as angiodema (severe swelling of the face, neck, and lips that interferes with speaking, swallowing, and breathing) or hives, stop taking Doryx at once and seek immediate medical attention. Because Doryx may make birth control pills less effective, ask your doctor if you should use an alternate form of birth control while taking this medication.

Possible Side Effects:
Bulging forehead in infants, headache, diarrhea, heightened sensitivity to light, difficulty swallowing, vomiting, discolored teeth in children, appetite loss, tongue inflammation, nausea, rash, and rectal itching.

Possible Drug Interactions:
Check with your doctor before taking Doryx along with other drugs. Doryx may interact with: antacids, barbiturates, bismuth subsalicylate (Pepto-Bismol), blood-thinning medications, carbamazepine (Tegretol), oral contraceptives, penicillin, phenytoin (Dilantin), and sodium bicarbonate.

Who Should Not Take This Drug:
Children under the age of eight and women in the second half of pregnancy should not take this drug, as it causes the discoloration of developing teeth. Because Doryx passes into breast milk, it should also be avoided if you are breast-feeding. Always tell your doctor about any medical conditions that you have. Doryx should be used with caution (if at all) if you have asthma.

How to Take This Drug:
To prevent throat irritation, take Doryx with a full glass of water. If it irritates your stomach, take it with milk or food.

What to Do If You Miss a Dose:
Take it as soon as you remember. If it is almost time for the next dose, take the one you missed, and take the remaining doses at even intervals throughout the rest of the day. Then return to your regular schedule.

Generic Name: Erythromycin
Brand Names: E.E.S., E-Mycin, ERYC, Ery-Tab, Erythrocin, Ilosone, and PCE

Erythromycin is a macrolide antibiotic with a long track record for safety. Before taking this drug, inform your doctor if you have ever experienced an allergic reaction to it in the past, or to similar antibiotics such as Biaxin or Zithromax. In such cases, a different antibiotic can be prescribed.

Caution:

If your doctor prescribes this drug and you experience symptoms such as severe or prolonged diarrhea or yellowing of the skin and eyes, stop taking erythromycin at once and seek immediate medical attention.

Possible Side Effects:

Nausea, vomiting, stomach cramps, diarrhea, colitis, appetite loss, skin rash, hairy tongue, rectal itching, and vaginal irritation.

Possible Drug Interactions:

Consult your doctor before combining erythromycin with other drugs. Erythromycin may interact with: antacids, blood-thinning drugs, bromocriptine (Parlodel), carbamazepine (Tegretol), cisapride (Propulsid), cyclosporine (Neoral and Sandimmune), digoxin (Lanoxin), disopyramide (Norpace), hexobarbital, lovastatin (Mevacor), phenytoin (Dilantin) and other seizure medications, tacrolimus (Prograf), triazolam (Halcion), ergot-containing drugs, and theophylline drugs.

Who Should Not Take This Drug:

Inform your doctor if you are or think you may be pregnant, or if you are breast-feeding; only he or she can determine if it is safe for you to take erythromycin. Also tell your doctor about any other medical conditions that you have. Erythromycin should be used with caution if you have liver disease. Do not take this drug if you have experienced a previous allergic reaction to it.

How to Take This Drug:

Consult your doctor for instructions.

What to Do If You Miss a Dose:
Take it as soon as you remember. If it is almost time for the next dose, take the one you missed, and take the remaining doses at even intervals throughout the rest of the day. Then return to your regular schedule.

Generic Name: Trimethoprim-sulfamethoxazole
Brand Names: Bactrim, Cotrim, and Septra
Also known as TMP-SMX, this combination drug is effective in many medical situations in which other drugs are not. Before taking TMP-SMX, inform your doctor if you have ever experienced an allergic reaction to either of its two components or to sulfa drugs.

Caution:
Sulfamethoxazole belongs to a group of medications called sulfonamides or sulfa drugs. Rare but potentially fatal reactions to sulfa drugs include toxic epidural necrolysis (also known as Stevens-Johnson syndrome, a life-threatening condition in which the skin blisters and peels off), severe liver damage, and blood and bone marrow disorders. Notify your doctor at once if you experience symptoms such as blood in your urine, any unusual bleeding or bruising, severe diarrhea, dizziness, confusion, extreme fatigue, fever, pallor, rash, sore throat, or yellowing of the skin and eyes.

Possible Side Effects:
Nausea, vomiting, upset stomach, diarrhea, heightened sensitivity to light, appetite loss, skin rash, itching, and hives.

Possible Drug Interactions:
Check with your doctor before combining TMP-SMX with other drugs. This medication may interact with blood thinners, methotrexate (Rheumatrex), phenytoin (Dilantin), and water pills.

Who Should Not Take This Drug:
You should not take TMP-SMX if you are or think you may be pregnant, or if you are breast-feeding. This drug should be used with caution (if at all) if you have liver or kidney disease, malabsorption, severe allergies, asthma, or folic acid deficiency, or if you are an alcoholic or have poor nutritional status. Also inform your doctor about any other medical conditions that you have. TMP-SMX should be

used with caution in seniors, and is not appropriate for infants under two months. Do not take this drug if you have experienced a previous allergic reaction to either of its components.

How to Take This Drug:
This drug is usually taken twice a day.

What to Do If You Miss a Dose:
Take it as soon as you remember. If it is almost time for the next dose, take the one you missed, and take the remaining doses at even intervals throughout the rest of the day. Then return to your regular schedule.

Treatment for Moderate Disease
Moderate disease is more serious. For example, an affected person might experience ten days of nasal congestion with increasing fever and sinus tenderness that worsens when he or she bends over. For moderate sinusitis—and for mild sinusitis in adults who *have* taken antibiotics in the previous four to six weeks—doctors recommend either amoxicillin-clavulanate (Augmentin) or one of three fluoro-quinolone antibiotics: gatifloxacin (Tequin), levofloxacin (Levaquin), or moxifloxacin (Avelox). (See our discussion of the fluoroquinolone group below.) Alternatively, a physician might prescribe a combination of amoxicillin (Amoxil and Trimox) or clindamycin (Cleocin) for gram-positive coverage plus cefixime (Suprax) for gram-negative coverage.

Fluoroquinolone Antibiotics: gatifloxacin (Tequin), levofloxacin (Levaquin), moxifloxacin (Avelox)
These relatively new antibiotics are also known simply as quinolones. Before taking a fluoroquinolone, tell your doctor if you have experienced an allergic reaction to any of the drugs in this group, so an alternate antibiotic can be prescribed.

Caution:
The fluoroquinolones have been known to cause dangerous and sometimes fatal allergic reactions after a single dose. Stop taking medication at once and seek immediate medical attention if you experience symptoms such as severe swelling of the face, neck, and lips; difficulty speaking, swallowing, or breathing; a skin rash or hives. If you experience palpitations or severe diarrhea, call your doctor.

Possible Side Effects:
Heightened sensitivity to sunlight, dizziness, drowsiness, lightheadedness, restlessness, trouble sleeping, palpitations, nausea, vomiting, diarrhea, stomach pain, fainting spells, tendon problems, and vaginal inflammation.

Possible Drug Interactions:
Check with your doctor before combining fluoroquinolones with other drugs. They may interact with: antacids that contain aluminum or magnesium (such as Gelusil or Maalox), amiodarone (Cordarone), bepridil (Vascor), cisapride (Propulsid), disopyramide (Norpace), erythromycin (E-Mycin, etc.), iron supplements, pentamidine (Nebupent), phenothiazines, procainamide (Pronestyl), quinidine (Quinidex), sotalol (Sotocor), theophylline drugs, and tricyclic antidepressants.

Who Should Not Take This Drug:
You should not take fluoroquinolones if you are or think you may be pregnant, or if you are breast-feeding. These drugs are not recommended for children under the age of eighteen. They should be used with caution if you have brain or spinal cord disease, heart disease, an irregular heartbeat, or tendonitis. Also inform your doctor about any other medical conditions that you have. Do not take a fluoroquinolone antibiotic if you have previously experienced an allergic reaction to one of the drugs in this group.

How to Take This Drug:
Unlike many other antibiotics, the fluoroquinolones are usually taken once a day. They are best taken with a full glass of water, either with or without food. Do not take any fluoroquinolone with antacids that contain aluminum or magnesium.

What to Do If You Miss a Dose:
Take it as soon as you remember. Do not try to catch up by doubling doses.

Switch Therapy

If your symptoms are unchanged or worsen after three days of antibiotic therapy, your doctor will want to reevaluate your condition. Possible tests at this time include CT scanning, nasal endoscopy, and sinus aspiration for culture. Depending upon the results, your doctor may switch you to a different and, one hopes, more effective antibiotic.

Side Effects and Adverse Reactions

As you've seen above, the most common side effects of antibiotics are stomach upset and diarrhea. Taking antibiotics after a meal is one useful step you can take to help eliminate mild gastrointestinal discomfort. But the longer you take these drugs, the more apt side effects are to occur. Anytime antibiotics are administered for more than two weeks, your body is depleted of its normal intestinal flora, leading to problems such as diarrhea. To prevent this type of upset, include yogurt in your daily diet, or take a lactobacillus supplement. This replenishes beneficial intestinal flora.

In some cases, more serious adverse reactions develop. If you are allergic to an antibiotic, the most common reaction is a skin rash. However, in rare cases, a life-threatening anaphylactic reaction may occur. This involves difficulty breathing and a dangerous drop in blood pressure. Immediate medical attention must be sought. In the future, avoid not only that antibiotic but related antibiotics as well.

ARE YOU ALLERGIC TO PENICILLIN?

- Always inform your doctor if you are allergic to penicillin.
- Amoxicillin (Amoxil and Trimox) and amoxicillin-clavulanate (Augmentin) belong to the same class of antibiotics as penicillin. If you are allergic to penicillin, you should not take these drugs.
- Cephalosporins are relatives of penicillin, and up to 15 percent of those allergic to penicillin may also be allergic to these drugs.

Antibiotics and Sinusitis in Children

Treatment of children is similar to that of adults, but there are some notable exceptions. The fluoroquinolone antibiotics are not approved for anyone under the age of eighteen. Combination therapy can be used even if your child has been given antibiotics in the previous six weeks. In some cases, cefpodoxime proxetil (Vantin) and trimethoprim-sulfamethoxazole (Bactrim, Cotrim, and Septra) may be used in combination therapy. (Read in greater detail about sinusitis in children in chapter 8.)

Oral Decongestants

Oral decongestants shrink swollen nasal and sinus membranes by constricting blood vessels. This limits blood flow, which reduces mucosal swelling—making it possible for you to feel more comfortable and breathe more freely. The most common oral decongestants are pseudoephedrine and phenylephrine. These are common ingredients in many over-the-counter cold and cough remedies.

Unfortunately, decongestants also have many possible side effects. These include nervousness, dizziness, a rapid heart rate, and insomnia. Some people refer to side effects as "the jitters." If you have hypertension, even a slight increase in blood pressure can be harmful, so speak to your physician before taking this type of sinus remedy. Men with enlarged prostates should likewise steer clear of oral decongestants, as they can worsen urinary retention.

Pseudoephedrine
Over-the-counter brands that contain pseudoephedrine include Sudafed and Triaminic. Their most common side effects are agitation, irritability, and insomnia. Less common adverse reactions include a change in heartbeat, difficulty breathing, nausea, vomiting, sweating, trembling, and painful urination or urinary retention. If you experience any of these problems, stop taking medication that contains pseudoephedrine and call your doctor. These medications should be used with caution (if at all) by anyone who suffers from high blood pressure, heart disease, an enlarged prostate, diabetes, or an overactive thyroid condition. If you are also taking other drugs, consult your doctor or pharmacist about possible drug interactions.

Phenylephrine
Dimetane is one of the most popular over-the-counter brands that contain phenylephrine. The most common side effect of these drugs is a fast or pounding heartbeat. Less common adverse reactions include dizziness, nervousness, insomnia, headache, and dryness in the nose. If you experience any of these problems, stop taking medication that contains phenylephrine and call your doctor. These medications should not be taken by anyone who suffers from high blood pressure, heart disease, an enlarged prostate, diabetes, or an overactive thyroid condition. If you are also taking other drugs, consult your doctor or pharmacist about possible drug interactions.

Topical Decongestants

In some cases, you may benefit more from a decongestant nasal spray than from the oral medication. Topical decongestants include napha-zoline HCI (Privine), oxymetazoline HCI (Afrin), and xylometazoline HCI (Otrivin). Like oral decongestants, these are available on an over-the-counter basis. Topical decongestants provide more immediate relief and help speed up drainage. They can be safely used for three days. However, using them for longer than this can cause a dangerous rebound effect. When the decongestant wears off, congestion and stuffiness may return in an even more severe form, prompting you to turn once more to the spray. This condition is known as rhinitis medicamentosa. It can lead to a vicious cycle in which you become more and more dependent on the nasal spray for congestion relief.

Mucous Thinners

Guaifenesin is the primary mucous thinner in liquid over-the-counter remedies such as plain Robitussin and tablets such as Humibid LA. This drug works by thinning secretions, thus improving sinus drainage. Side effects are not common, but may include rash (such as hives), dizziness, headache, nausea, and vomiting. If you experience any of these problems, stop taking guaifenesin and call your doctor.

Steroid and Saline Sprays

Steroid nasal sprays—such as budesonide (Rhinocort), fluticasone (Flonase), mometasone (Nasonex), and triamcinolone (Nasacort)—reduce nasal and sinus swelling. Also referred to as topical or intra-nasal steroids, these medications are not particularly beneficial in the early stages of acute disease. They take time to work, and initial tissue swelling actually hinders the medication's ability to penetrate mucosal tissue. But after several days of antibiotic therapy, the anti-inflammatory action of steroid sprays can speed healing. In those who have recurrent acute disease, they are a good preventive measure because they lessen swelling in the osteomeatal unit. And since they come as a spray rather than a swallowable pill or capsule, there are fewer side effects. (While extremely beneficial in the treatment of chronic sinusitis, oral corticosteroids—with their numerous side effects—are rarely used in the treatment of acute sinusitis.)

Saline sprays may also help you breathe more easily and feel better overall. In cases of severe congestion, doctors even recommend using saline sprays prior to steroid sprays in order to prevent nasal irritation or stinging. Saline clears the sinuses of thickened secretions and crusty debris, and may improve mucociliary transport and decrease viscosity of secretions. While commercial saline sprays are available over-the-counter, you can also make your own nasal irrigation rinse with a quart of tap or bottled water; two to three teaspoons of salt (with no iodine or other additives); and a teaspoon of baking soda. This can be stored for up to a week at room temperature; shake before using. Spray saline into each nostril while closing off the other nostril and simultaneously inhaling.

ANABOLIC STEROIDS VERSUS CORTICOSTEROIDS

Although the term *steroids* is loosely applied to both, corticosteroids and anabolic steroids are two entirely different medications. Corticosteroids are extremely useful medications in the treatment of a variety of inflammatory disorders, while anabolic steroids are dangerous synthetic derivatives of testosterone that athletes use to build muscle.

Topical Anticholinergics

These sprays—such as Atrovent Nasal Spray 0.03% (ipratropium bromide)—are used for the relief of runny nose (rhinorrhea). The usual dosage is two sprays per nostril two to three times a day. Common and relatively harmless side effects of Atrovent are nasal drying and crusting. Also beware of rare but extremely serious hypersensitivity reactions such as severe swelling of the face, neck, and lips; difficulty speaking, swallowing, or breathing; and a skin rash or hives. Do not use this drug if you are allergic to atropine, or if you have narrow-angle glaucoma, bladder problems, or prostate problems.

Antihistamines Are Generally Not Recommended

Although there is no evidence that they are effective in treating acute sinusitis, many people turn to over-the-counter or prescription antihistamines for relief. But antihistamines are meant to treat allergies, not sinusitis. Because they work by blocking the body's release of the mediator histamine, antihistamines are an appropriate treatment only when sinusitis is associated with allergies. (Read more about antihistamines later in this chapter, under "Allergy Medications.")

CHRONIC SINUSITIS

A key distinction between acute and chronic sinus disease lies in the types of organisms involved. Anaerobes—stubborn bacteria that live and grow in the absence of oxygen—are more commonly detected in chronic sinusitis, although it is unclear whether this is a cause or an effect of the disease. In addition, multiple organisms are seen more frequently than in acute infections. But in spite of our better understanding of chronic disease (including its immune and inflammatory factors), as well as dramatic technical advances in diagnosis and surgical treatment, this remains a complex and challenging disorder to manage. Because there is still no one definitive surgical cure, optimal treatment often combines medical and surgical approaches. Doctors recommend antibiotics (the same ones as for acute disease), corticosteroids, decongestants, mucous thinners, and topical anticholinergics. As with acute disease, antihistamines are recommended only when chronic sinusitis is associated with allergies. Similarly, mast cell stabilizers should be used only when allergies are a complicating factor.

Antibiotics

Most doctors continue to believe that antibiotics play an important role in the treatment of chronic sinusitis. Although there is some controversy surrounding the length of therapy, the consensus is that three to six weeks is optimal. Stubborn cases, of course, require longer courses of antibiotics. When chronic disease is caused by fungi, antibiotics are not an appropriate treatment.

TAKE ANTIBIOTICS EXACTLY AS PRESCRIBED BY YOUR DOCTOR
Many people discontinue medication once they feel better. This is a mistake, for stopping too soon can result in a more stubborn and intractable infection. Always take antibiotics exactly as your physician instructs, including the number of days and the number of times each day prescribed.

Taking a Nasal Culture

Analysis of a nasal culture enables your doctor to choose an antibiotic that will be effective against your particular infection. A sample secretion is usually obtained in the course of a nasal endoscopy performed in your physician's office. Endoscopy has largely come to replace older and more painful invasive procedures such as antral puncture. It is performed using a rigid, rodlike fiberoptic instrument that your doctor uses to probe inside your nose and sinuses. Before the procedure, you will be given a local anesthetic and decongestant to lessen discomfort. Unfortunately, simply swabbing the nose does not provide a sufficiently reliable sample.

Side Effects and Adverse Reactions

As mentioned earlier, the most common side effect of antibiotics is stomach discomfort. In order to prevent this problem, take your medication after a meal. Any long-term use also increases the risk of diarrhea and oral or vaginal yeast infections. Eating yogurt with active cultures on a daily basis or taking acidophilus capsules may protect against these reactions. Once available primarily at health food stores, acidophilus supplements are sold today at most pharmacies. If you experience symptoms such as severe nausea and vomiting, stop taking your medication at once and contact your physician for further advice. Always inform your doctor if you have allergies to any drugs.

BEWARE OF DRUG INTERACTIONS

In order to avoid dangerous interactions, always inform both your doctor and your pharmacist of all prescription drugs, over-the-counter medications, vitamins, and complementary remedies that you are taking.

Steroids

Also known as corticosteroids or glucocorticoids, these powerful anti-inflammatory medications are among the most useful drugs in the treatment of chronic sinusitis. Because we now understand chronic disease to have important immune and inflammatory as well as infectious components, medications such as steroids have assumed a primary role in the treatment of this disorder. Because they reduce inflammation and swelling of mucous membranes, steroids are also beneficial in the treatment of allergies and asthma. These drugs are available in intra-nasal, oral, inhaled, and injectable form. (Inhaled steroids breathed in through the mouth are for asthma, while injections are reserved for severe inflammatory reactions.)

Steroid Sprays

Nasal steroid sprays are valuable in chronic as well as acute disease. In addition to shrinking swollen mucous membranes, these sprays may reduce nasal polyps. In contrast to the oral medication, steroid sprays have minimal side effects. Still, they must be properly used, with medication directed into the nasal cavity rather than onto the nasal septum (the wall dividing the two sides of the nose). Otherwise, long-term use can lead to septum damage or even perforation. If you have any questions, ask your doctor to show you the proper way to use steroid sprays. Other possible side effects include glaucoma, cataracts, atrophic rhinitis, and suppression of hormone secretions by the adrenal glands. Because of these potential problems, you should be periodically monitored while taking this medication on a long-term basis.

Oral Steroids

Since steroids are associated with serious side effects, topical forms (rather than pills or capsules that you swallow) are the safest method of delivery. When oral medication is prescribed, doctors generally begin with the lowest possible dose and gradually taper it down-ward. Short bursts of seven to ten days usually cause minimal if any side effects. If you require long-term treatment for a chronic problem, low doses are preferable, as they are associated with fewer complications. Because steroids are so effective, sometimes only two weeks of therapy can make a significant difference in a difficult chronic case.

ORAL STEROIDS FOR CHRONIC SINUSITIS

Since it is relatively inexpensive, prednisone (Deltasone) is the most commonly prescribed oral steroid. Others include betamethasone (Celestone), dexamethasone (Decadron), and methylprednisolone (Medrol). A description of what you can expect when you take one of these medications is on the next page.

Oral Steroids: Betamethasone (Celestone), dexamethasone (Decadron), methylprednisolone (Medrol), prednisone (Deltasone)
Steroids are powerful drugs used to reduce inflammation.

Caution:
Steroids have many serious side effects. They should be taken only when their benefits clearly outweigh their risks.

Possible Side Effects:
Weight gain, fluid retention, bloating, rounding of the face, thinning of the skin, changes in appetite, stomach upset, ulcers, muscle weakness, easy bruising, stunted growth, reduced immunity, osteoporosis, hypertension, and cataracts.

Possible Drug Interactions:
Check with your doctor before combining steroids with other drugs. They may interact with: antacids, barbiturates, carbamazepine (Tegretol), cyclosporine (Neoral and Sandimmune), digitalis, griseofulvin (Fulvicin), mitotane (Lysodren), phenylbutazone (Butazolidin), phenytoin (Dilantin), primidone (Mysoline), rifampin (Rifadin), oral diabetes medications, diuretics, and immunizations.

Who Should Not Take These Drugs:
You should not take steroids if you are or think you may be pregnant, or if you are breast-feeding. These drugs are not recommended for long-term use in children, because they may stunt youngsters' growth. Seniors may be more likely to develop side effects from steroid use. Steroids should be used with caution (if at all) if you have immune problems, hypertension, diabetes, bleeding disorders, peptic ulcer disease, glaucoma, osteoporosis, a systemic fungal infection, ocular herpes simplex, liver disease, high cholesterol, tuberculosis, or recent surgery. Also inform your doctor about any other medical conditions that you have. You should not take steroids if you have previously experienced an allergic reaction to a steroid drug.

How to Take These Drugs:
Take steroids with food to prevent stomach upset.

What to Do If You Miss a Dose:
Take it as soon as you remember. Do not try to catch up by doubling doses.

Steroids Fight Inflammation

Steroids are chemical derivatives of a human hormone produced by your body's adrenal gland. Especially when taken orally, they dramatically reduce the body's levels of basophils, eosinophils, and monocytes, cells that are closely involved in inflammation. Eosinophils in particular play a major role in chronic sinusitis. By reducing their number, movement, and survival time, steroids inhibit the release of inflammatory substances such as histamine.

Beware of Serious Side Effects

Helpful as steroids can be in controlling dangerous inflammation, their use comes at a price. Long-term use of oral steroids can impede the body's own ability to produce essential adrenal hormones and increases the risk of serious health problems such as osteoporosis, hypertension, and cataracts. Other adverse effects include weight gain, fluid retention, bloating, rounding of the face, thinning of the skin, stomach upset, ulcers, muscle weakness, easy bruising, stunted growth, and reduced immunity. Steroids should be used with caution in people who have immune problems, hypertension, diabetes, bleeding disorders, peptic ulcer disease, glaucoma, or osteoporosis. They should not be used if you are hypersensitive to steroids, if you have a systemic fungal infection, or if you have ocular herpes simplex.

Decongestants

These drugs too are important in the treatment of chronic as well as acute disease. By constricting blood supply to nasal mucosa, decongestants result in less swelling, a decreased volume of blood in the sinuses, and reduced resistance to nasal airflow. In chronic sinusitis, these medications are sometimes prescribed for long periods of time. However, this can result in side effects such as insomnia, and special care must be taken with individuals who have health problems such as hypertension or enlarged prostates. Decongestant nasal sprays take effect more quickly and are more useful overall; they also have fewer side effects than oral decongestants. However, if used for longer than three days, they have a dangerous rebound effect.

Other Medications for Chronic Sinusitis

A variety of other medications are also used to fight chronic sinusitis. Some are very helpful, while others are not so beneficial. Guaifenesin—

a safe and effective drug found in over-the-counter brands such as plain Robitussin—efficiently thins secretions and improves sinus drainage in chronic sinusitis. Topical intranasal anticholinergics—such as Atrovent Nasal Spray 0.03%—relieve runny noses. Intranasal cromolyn sodium—for example, Nasalcrom—can be helpful if there is an allergic component. Mast cell stabilizers such as Nasalcrom are considered very safe and are available without a prescription. Because they are free from the serious side effects associated with topical corticosteroids, these drugs are an especially attractive alternative for children. Treatment should begin two or three weeks before the onset of allergy season and continue throughout its duration. Antihistamines are appropriate only if you simultaneously suffer from chronic sinusitis *and* allergies, with symptoms such as a runny nose, sneezing, and itching.

MEDICATIONS FOR COMPLICATIONS

Serious complications from sinusitis can cause blindness or even death. Since the advent of antibiotics, complications have fortunately become much less frequent. Still, when they occur, eye and brain problems—the two most severe forms of sinusitis complications—require early and aggressive intervention.

Eye Complications

Orbital, or eye, complications almost invariably require hospitalization for further evaluation and treatment. Since bacteria (most frequently, *Hemophilus influenzae*, *Moraxella catarrhalis*, and *Streptococcus pyogenes* or *S. pneumoniae*) are the usual cause of orbital infection, antibiotics are the mainstay of treatment. Your physician may also prescribe topical nasal vasoconstrictors such as Afrin—medications that relieve nasal congestion and improve breathing. Steroids are not recommended because of potential complications. Although antibiotic therapy is usually successful in the treatment of the less serious forms of orbital complications—periorbital cellulitis and orbital cellulitis—surgery is often required in more severe cases.

Brain Complications

Like eye problems, brain complications are very serious and require hospitalization. Most intracranial complications require a hospital stay of approximately a month. Once you are admitted to the hospital, you will be placed on intravenous antibiotics that penetrate the central nervous system. Since eight out of ten brain complications cause seizures, you will also be given anticonvulsant medications. In cases of severe brain swelling, steroids are recommended. Some intracranial complications—notably meningitis—are treated mainly with medications. However, many others require surgical intervention.

MEDICATIONS FOR UNDERLYING CONDITIONS

It is vital to control any underlying conditions that lead to sinusitis. Otherwise, you may end up with sinus infection after sinus infection. Medications are a key element of treatment.

Cold Medications

Many different cold and cough mixtures exist to treat any possible combination of symptoms. The dilemma is which, if any, to use. You must make this choice according to your own needs and responses. Make it a point to read labels—what are the ingredients of the remedy you are purchasing? Many contain ingredients that you do not require. For instance, if your cold or sinusitis is nonallergic, there is no reason to subject yourself to the side effects of a remedy that includes an antihistamine. Also be on the alert for combinations of multisymptom drugs that contain analgesics. Since these are a component of so many over-the-counter cold and sinus medications, you might accidentally take more acetaminophen or aspirin than you intended—first as part of a general combination remedy, and then by taking a pill for a headache or fever.

The most common drugs in cold remedies are discussed below.

Decongestants

These drugs shrink swollen nasal membranes by constricting blood vessels. If you have a cold or flu, medications such as Sudafed can help relieve your congestion, thus allowing you to breathe freely and possibly offering some protection against secondary sinus infections. Possible side effects include nervousness, dizziness, a rapid heart rate, and insomnia. Tell your physician if you have an underlying condition such as hypertension or an enlarged prostate. If you choose a decongestant spray, use it exactly as directed and for no longer than three days, in order to prevent a rebound effect. (See page 97 for a more detailed discussion of decongestants.)

Cough Suppressants

These medications calm the irritating tickle that leads to unnecessary coughs. Dextromethorphan is the most common nonnarcotic cough suppressant. While it suppresses unproductive coughs caused by irritation, this drug does not suppress the useful, productive coughs that are required to clear phlegm. Dextromethorphan is very effective and has no side effects when taken in normal doses. (Codeine is also an efficient cough suppressant, but it is a powerful narcotic and not available in over-the-counter preparations.) Cough and cold remedies that contain dextromethorphan include brands such as Contac, Nyquil, and Robitussin. Less common or rare adverse reactions include confusion, dizziness, excitement, nervousness, drowsiness, rash, diarrhea, nausea, and vomiting. If you experience any of these problems, discontinue use and contact your doctor.

Mucous Thinners

Drugs such as guaifenesin—by far the most common mucous thinner, or expectorant—loosen phlegm and help the cough lift it out of bronchial tubes. They are believed to work by increasing mucous output, resulting in thinner mucus that is easier for cilia to sweep through the respiratory tract. Brands with this drug include plain Robitussin liquid and Humibid LA. No serious side effects have been reported from taking guaifenesin, but see page 98 for possible side effects.

Analgesics

These drugs control fever and provide pain relief. Aspirin-free acetaminophen is one of the most popular pain relievers for cold and sinus sufferers. However, although most of us think nothing of taking acetaminophen (the active ingredient in Tylenol) for a cold or sinus headache, even this basic over-the-counter medication must be used correctly in order for it to be safe as well as effective. When taken in excess, in conjunction with alcohol, or by people with preexisting liver or kidney problems, acetaminophen can cause liver and kidney damage. Aspirin, also very effective in reducing pain and fever, has a long and impressive safety record. Unlike acetaminophen, it also has an impact on inflammation. Nonetheless, aspirin can cause gastrointestinal (GI) bleeding if taken too often or in excess. Children and adolescents should never be given aspirin, which is associated with a rare but life-threatening childhood condition known as Reye's syndrome. NSAIDs (nonsteroidal anti-inflammatory drugs) such as ibuprofen (the active ingredient in Advil and Motrin) are similar to aspirin in their ability to relieve pain, fever, and inflammation, but also in their tendency to promote GI bleeding. For this reason, neither aspirin nor NSAIDs should be taken for ten days to two weeks prior to any surgery.

Antihistamines

Once again: these drugs are not for colds, any more than they are for sinusitis. Antihistamines relieve the runny nose, sneezing, and itching of allergies—they do not in general help nasal blockage. Nevertheless, many combination cold medications on the market contain antihistamines. If you only have a cold, *do not* take these medications. Consider them only if you suffer from both allergies and a cold.

ANTIBIOTICS ARE NOT FOR COLDS

When cold symptoms persist for longer than ten days, you may have developed a secondary bacterial infection such as sinusitis. Your physician will most likely prescribe antibiotics for this problem. But there is a very big difference between the treatment of colds and that of sinusitis. Colds are caused by viruses. Antibiotics have no impact on viruses and should not be prescribed for them. Much as we yearn for a magic pill to make us feel better when we are suffering from a cold, it is useless—and potentially even harmful—to take antibiotics for viral infection. Antibiotics come into play only when a cold causes a secondary bacterial infection. (To review the overuse of antibiotics in greater detail, turn to page 6.)

Allergy Medications

Several groups of medicines can relieve allergic symptoms and control the inflammation associated with chronic allergies.

Antihistamines

In the course of this chapter, we've talked about what conditions antihistamines are *not* meant for, such as colds and simple, nonallergic sinusitis. But antihistamines *can and often do* play a crucial role in controlling the runny noses, itchy eyes, and sneezing of allergies.

These medications work by blocking histamine, a substance normally released in small amounts by the body's mast cells, but in substantial amounts during allergic reactions. Of course, like all medications, antihistamines have side effects—and, in this case, the possible side effects are unpredictable and widely variable. Some individuals become drowsy after taking an antihistamine, while others experience nervousness and insomnia. Children who are given them may become nervous and agitated.

There are two important categories of antihistamines. Older, first-generation antihistamines—such as those found in over-the-counter Benadryl—cross from the bloodstream into the brain, where they produce drowsiness. Newer, second-generation antihistamines, which as of now are available by prescription only, do not cross the blood-brain barrier. This means that they are either nonsedating (Allegra, Claritin, and Clarinex) or have only mild sedative effects (Astelin and Zyrtec). These drugs can be extremely beneficial, but again, you must be careful of their side effects.

ANTIHISTAMINES FOR ALLERGIES

Older antihistamines:

Brompheniramine (Dimetane and generics)
Chlorpheniramine (Chlor-Trimeton and generics)
Clemastine (Tavist-1 and generics)
Diphenhydramine (Benadryl and generics)

Newer nondrowsy antihistamines:

Fexofenadine (Allegra)
Loratadine (Claritin)
Desloratadine (Clarinex)

Newer semidrowsy antihistamines:

Azelastine (Astelin)
Cetirizine (Zyrtec)

Other Medications for Allergies

In addition to antihistamines, a variety of other drugs are often deployed against allergies. For example, decongestants are taken to relieve nasal congestion by constricting blood vessels in the mucous membranes. Corticosteroids may also be beneficial—but their risks versus benefits must be carefully weighed. Cromolyn sodium (Nasalcrom)—a nonsteroidal nasal spray—is a safe and effective anti-inflammatory drug that is now available over-the-counter. Treatment should begin two or three weeks before the onset of allergy season and continue throughout its duration. Finally, immunotherapy—which consists of allergy or desensitizing shots—prevents allergic reactions by reducing the number of eosinophils and T cells. The shots involve injecting very small but gradually increasing amounts of an allergen over a period of weeks or months. Not everyone benefits from immunotherapy, and there is also a small risk of a life-threatening allergic reaction known as anaphylaxis. This emergency condition, which involves a sharp drop in blood pressure and difficulty breathing, must be treated promptly with an epinephrine injection.

Asthma Medications

There are basically two types of asthma medications. Anti-inflammatory drugs prevent asthma symptoms, while bronchodilators are used to manage asthmatic episodes or attacks.

Anti-inflammatory drugs

These medications are taken to *prevent* the symptoms of asthma. Anti-inflammatory drugs stabilize the mast cells that release inflammatory chemicals when exposed to triggers. When there is less inflammation in the airways, there are fewer asthmatic episodes and a reduced risk of permanent lung damage due to uncontrolled inflammation. Inhaled steroids and cromolyn sodium are examples of anti-inflammatory medications.

Bronchodilators

These drugs are used to *control* symptoms once they occur. Bronchodilators work by quickly opening blocked airways. They relax the muscles around airways, which allows air to move more freely in and out of the lungs. Bronchodilators are usually taken in inhaled form, through metered-dose inhalers or nebulizers, to relieve the shortness of breath, tight chest, coughing, and wheezing of an asthma attack. They are breathed in through the mouth. Examples of bronchodilators include albuterol (Proventil), metaproterenol (Alupent), salmeterol

(Serevent), terbutaline (Brethine), and theophylline drugs (Quibron-T/SR, Slo-Bid, T-Phyl, Theochron, Theo-Dur, Uni-Dur, and Uniphyl).

WHEN MEDICINE ALONE IS NOT ENOUGH

In mild to moderate acute sinusitis, medication—along with other strategies, such as maintaining a healthy lifestyle and avoiding allergens and pollutants—is usually sufficient. On the other hand, tenacious and drug-resistant cases of chronic or recurrent acute sinusitis sometimes demand surgical intervention. In the next chapter, you will learn more about today's less invasive approach to sinus surgery.

CHAPTER 7

When Surgery Is Necessary

Like medication, surgery plays a key role in the treatment of sinus disease. Over the course of the last two decades, remarkable advances have taken place in intranasal surgery, as newer and less invasive techniques have gradually come to supersede traditional surgery. Nevertheless, surgery is a serious proposition that should be considered only when all other forms of medical treatment have been exhausted.

THE INDICATIONS FOR SURGERY

Because chronic sinus disease has so many different underlying causes, there are likewise many different approaches to treatment. These range from medications—such as extended courses of more than one antibiotic for infection, and allergy treatment when appropriate—to lifestyle changes—for example, avoiding the triggers of allergies or quitting your job in a "sick building" (see page 56). Often these measures alone are sufficient to control sinus disease. But in chronic or acute recurrent cases that fail to respond to these actions, surgery represents another option.

Sinus surgery is performed for a variety of reasons. In some cases, it is necessary to clean and drain the sinuses. Other times, an operation is required to reopen or enlarge the natural openings of the sinuses to allow drainage and ventilation. Procedures may also be performed to remove an obstructive growth, such as a polyp, tumor, or cyst. Absolute indications for surgery include extensive mucoceles (swollen sacs or cavities filled with mucus) or mucopyceles (infected mucoceles), allergic or invasive fungal disease, suspected tumors, and the development of serious eye or brain complications.

Interestingly, doctors consider chronic and recurrent acute sinusitis as only relative indications for surgery. While some people with these conditions benefit from surgery, this type of intervention is by no means uniformly successful, nor is it required in every case. Surgery is elective and should be postponed until you have tried all the more-conservative forms of medical therapy, and until even lifestyle changes have proven ineffective.

INDICATIONS FOR SURGERY

- Mucoceles (swollen sacs or cavities filled with mucus) or mucopyceles (infected mucoceles)
- Fungal sinusitis
- Possible malignancy
- The development of serious eye or brain complications, such as orbital cellulitis, orbital abscess, brain abscess, meningitis, or cavernous sinus thrombosis

MAKING THE DECISION

In spite of impressive technological advances, surgery is no walk in the park. Any type of surgery is still a big deal and carries certain inherent risks (for example, infection, or that rare slip of an instrument that can lead to a perforation). So how do you make the decision whether or not to have surgery? As we mentioned above, sometimes you have no choice. Unusually severe complications—such as those that affect the eyes or brain—unequivocally call for prompt intervention. Obstructions such as polyps are relative—but not absolute—indications for surgery. Some doctors feel that asymptomatic polyps should be monitored, but not necessarily surgically removed; others believe that they should at least be biopsied, to see whether or not they are cancerous or precancerous. And once you travel beyond these parameters and enter the murky world inhabited by the vast majority of chronic sinusitis sufferers, the decision becomes even less clear-cut.

Most people considering surgery have chronic sinusitis that is not life-threatening. On the other hand, even though it's not going to kill you, persistent pain and inflammation can leave you in extreme physical discomfort and have a negative impact on your overall quality of life. Perhaps you always feel as if you have a cold, are tired and depressed, or are missing so many days of work that you are in danger of losing your job. People try many different strategies to fight these and other manifestations of chronic sinusitis. You may have taken multiple courses of antibiotics, as well as a battery of other medications, including decongestants, steroids, and mucous thinners. If your problem is related to allergies or other underlying medical conditions, by now you've done your best to address and control them. You've installed a humidifier in your dry bedroom, and a dehumidifier in your damp basement. In frustration, many people also turn to alternative treatment such as herbs or homeopathic remedies. (Read more about these in chapter 10.) It is only when all else fails, and symptoms persist in spite of your best efforts, that you should begin to think about surgery.

The reality, however, is that surgery is not a magic bullet for most chronic sinus sufferers. It is best considered as an adjunct to medical therapy. If chronic inflammation is severe, it may take months—or even years—after surgery to settle down. It is also important to keep in mind that surgery is not uniformly successful. Generally speaking, individuals with relatively mild disease or a specific localized problem (such as a mucocele) report the best postsurgical results. People with severe, chronic pain and inflammation may obtain relief—but then again, they may not. For all these reasons, it is essential to explore at length with your physician all the possible risks and benefits before making a joint decision about sinus surgery. It is important to have realistic expectations about what surgery can and cannot—and might and might not—achieve.

Ask the Right Questions

As you look into whether surgery is your best option, there are a number of questions to ask and factors to consider. They include the following:

Is this an emergency situation? Or do you have other options?

What other treatments have you tried? Has your doctor prescribed a variety of antibiotics? How many courses of antibiotics have you taken?

What other medications have you tried?

Have you been examined for other, underlying conditions that may contribute to sinus disease? If you have been diagnosed with a medical condition such as allergies or reflux, have you been optimally treated for this problem?

Are there any factors in your home or work environment that are aggravating your symptoms? If so, have you made every possible effort to correct them?

Do you find that your symptoms are worse at certain times of year?

Do you smoke?

Have you consulted a specialist, such as an otolaryngologist?

What tests have you undergone? Nasal endoscopy? CT scanning? MRI? Do the results show any clear evidence of disease? Do they show any structural abnormalities (such as a badly deviated septum) or an obstruction (such as a polyp or cyst)?

Have you had your adenoids removed?

Have you had any recent dental work? When was your last dental checkup?

Have you had previous sinus surgery?

How is chronic sinusitis affecting your quality of life?

How do you sleep at night? Do you suffer from sleep apnea? Do you find yourself tired and sluggish during the day? Do you take daytime naps?

Do you suffer from headaches? How often? Would you rate their pain as mild, moderate, or severe?

Do you find yourself feeling anxious or depressed? Are you unusually irritable with other people?

Has sinusitis affected your sense of smell? Your sense of taste?

How many days of work have you missed this year?

DIAGNOSTIC EVALUATION FOR SURGERY

Certain tests are critical in determining whether or not surgery is recommended. In particular, nasal endoscopy and high-resolution CT (computerized tomography) imaging can detect sinus problems that are not readily identifiable by any other means. Not very long ago, X rays were routinely used for diagnosing sinus disease and indicating when surgery was necessary. However, the inaccurateness of this technique led to both overdiagnosis and underdiagnosis. X rays are particularly inadequate in visualizing the structures of the osteomeatal unit, which play a key role in inflammatory sinus disease (see page 73).

In contrast, nasal endoscopy allows doctors to accurately assess the OMU for local infection or anatomic defects that interfere with ventilation and mucociliary clearance. One of the greatest advances in the diagnosis of sinusitis, this test is performed with the aid of a rigid, rodlike fiberoptic instrument that the doctor uses to look inside your nose and sinuses. An endoscope can also be used to remove a sample of mucus to culture in the laboratory; this will determine which bacteria or other microorganism is responsible for your symptoms. Before endoscopy, you will be given a local anesthetic and decongestant to lessen any discomfort. If the procedure reveals findings such as purulence and blockage of the osteomeatal unit, your doctor will diagnose sinusitis and may go on to order CT scanning.

CT scanning—the gold standard of imaging studies for sinus disease—can detect mucosal changes deeper in the OMU that are beyond the reach of endoscopy. CT provides a clear display of the sinuses not afforded by any other imaging technique. It is particularly effective in detecting bony abnormalities that contribute to sinus disease but can be surgically corrected. CT can also indicate the extent of disease. Coronal CT scanning is commonly recommended in people who have complications and those for whom surgery is being considered. However, CT imaging should not be the sole determinant of surgery, because mucosal thickening also typically occurs with viral upper respiratory infections. Mucosal changes can also be seen in asymptomatic patients. This can lead to overdiagnosis and overtreatment. Consequently, surgery is reserved for people who have symptoms of chronic sinusitis, with evidence on endoscopy and CT scan, and who have failed to respond to various kinds of nonsurgical med-

---

IS PAIN AN INDICATION FOR SURGERY?

When you experience chronic sinus headaches and pain, you may believe that surgery is the answer. In some cases, this is true. For example, if you typically have severe pain with pressure changes during air travel, you may have a sinus obstruction. But other times, pain is not due to sinus disease. Only careful evaluation with nasal endoscopy and CT scanning can determine whether or not surgery is warranted.

ical treatment. Surgery is scheduled when you and your doctor jointly decide that medical management is not providing sufficient relief of your symptoms.

SINUS SURGERY

Functional endoscopic sinus surgery (FESS) has become the method of choice in surgery for sinus disease. This procedure is less invasive than conventional surgery, gets better results, and complications are rare. Nine out of ten endoscopic operations result in significant improvement.

Looking Back

Only twenty years ago, sinus surgery was a bloody and traumatic experience. External incisions were the rule, more tissue was removed, and afterward the nose was usually packed with bandages. Preendoscopy, surgeons made incisions in the gums under the upper lip or through slits in the face to gain access to the sinuses. Operations took hours and required a hospital stay and extensive recovery period. Today, all that has changed, thanks to functional endoscopic sinus surgery. In this procedure, no external incision is required, and less tissue is removed with better results. The operations are short, and unless there are complications, you can go home the same day and get back to work in several days.

Functional Endoscopic Sinus Surgery (FESS)

The goals of functional endoscopic sinus surgery are to promote better sinus drainage and repair problems while removing as little tissue as possible. FESS allows your surgeon to see inside your sinuses and to accurately assess even small changes in the OMU that can impede ventilation and mucociliary clearance of the frontal, ethmoid, and maxillary sinuses. This approach is best when extensive sinus disease is caused by a localized problem, such as a mass that the doctor can see and remove through the endoscope. For example, a mucocele that causes obstruction of the frontal sinus is ideally treated with endoscopic surgery. Complete removal of a fungal ball from a maxillary sinus can likewise cure a nasty case of noninvasive fungal sinusitis. The mass is simply scooped up and suctioned out through the endoscope using a tiny tool that looks very much like a spoon.

Preparing for Surgery

Before surgery, your doctor may prescribe a course of antibiotics for one to three weeks. Drug selection is commonly based on culture results. Your physician may also prescribe oral steroids to shrink polyps or stabilize hyperreactive mucous membranes. This can reduce the risk of bleeding during surgery. In most cases, a CT scan of your sinuses will be ordered. In addition, you must stop taking all aspirin compounds and nonsteroidal anti-inflammatory drugs (such as Advil and Motrin) two to three weeks prior to surgery—these are associated with an increased risk of bleeding. Also stop taking alternative remedies for two to three weeks—these may cause problems such as bleeding, prolonged anesthetic effects, delay in waking, or blood pressure fluctuations. Finally, in order to prevent stomach contents from entering your lungs during surgery (aspiration), your doctor will instruct you to not to eat or drink for eight hours before surgery.

Powered Instrumentation

In recent years, powered instruments—in particular, microdebriders—have become common in FESS. Microdebriders are precise cutting instruments that were originally employed in oral and orthopedic surgery. They provide greater safety in sinus surgery along with decreased trauma to normal tissue. Powered instruments are used to precisely remove soft tissue ranging from tiny polyps to large tumors, as well as fine bony fragments. All powered instruments have a number of the same features: a suction-dependent motorized handpiece; a rotating inner cannula housed inside a fixed outer cannula; a cutting surface at the lateral aspect of the distal tip; and the ability to draw tissue into the port, shear it off, and evacuate it from the surgical field.

During the Procedure

Functional endoscopic sinus surgery typically lasts between one and two and a half hours. After appropriate anesthesia—which may be local with sedation or general anesthesia—the surgeon inserts a tube called a fiberoptic nasal endoscope into the patient's nostril. This permits detailed examination and treatment of the nose and sinuses. The surgeon may work through the endoscope or may beam what it sees onto a video screen in the operating room. He or she then guides a delicate miniature tool through the endoscope. Using such tiny tools, the surgeon can enlarge a narrow sinus passage, drain an abscess, or remove diseased tissue or a bone that is blocking a passage. For instance, as he or she presses a foot pedal, a rotating blade on a microdebrider shears off unwanted tissue, which is immediately sucked into the tube. This controls current infection and promotes better future drainage to prevent recurrences.

In contrast to older, more extensive procedures, stripping membranes and exposing bone are strictly avoided during endoscopic surgery. To whatever extent possible, normal mucosal tissue is left undisturbed. Another change in surgery is that secondary openings are rarely created today to improve drainage—it has become clear that the cilia will inevitably direct mucus toward the original, primary openings, or ostia. At the close of the procedure, some surgeons pack the nose. Packing can be absorbable or nonabsorbable; nonabsorbable packing must be removed by the surgeon postoperatively in the office. In pediatric cases, absorbable packs are usually used.

Image-Guided Surgery

In some sinus surgery procedures, doctors use CT scanning to provide a kind of three-dimensional road map to the sinuses. This technique permits the surgeon to identify the position of his or her instruments in sinus passages and to coordinate it with their position on the CT scan present in the operating room. This correlation increases safety and efficiency in patients with extensive disease and complex anatomy. Image-guided surgery is especially important in difficult cases.

What to Expect Following Surgery

Most people experience only minor pain following endoscopic surgery. Once the anesthesia wears off, you can usually go home. An overnight stay is necessary only if you have complications such as bleeding and swelling, or if you have an accompanying medical problem (for example, asthma). Your doctor will recommend a liquid diet to begin with, gradually followed by solids as you can tolerate them. Avoid aspirin, NSAIDs (such as Advil or Motrin), and alternative remedies immediately after surgery because of the risk of bleeding.

Postsurgical treatment consists of daily nasal saline irrigation, antibiotics, and steroids. Your doctor will usually prescribe a two-week course of antibiotics, and intranasal steroid sprays for up to four months. However, if underlying sinus disease is extensive and involves bony osteitis, oral antibiotic therapy may continue for six weeks or longer. In some cases, intravenous antibiotics are required. Topical or oral decongestants may also be recommended. If your nose was packed with nonabsorbable packing during surgery, this will be removed on a subsequent office visit.

Weekly follow-up is generally advised for six weeks. At these appointments, your doctor will use a nasal endoscope to clean dried blood and mucus from sinus cavities. Before this procedure, you will be given a topical decongestant and a local anesthetic to make you more comfortable. Occasionally, follow-up surgery is necessary. Notify your doctor immediately if you experience symptoms such as excessive bleeding, fever, increased swelling and/or bulging of the face or eyelids, bulging of the eye, or loss of vision.

SMOKING AND FESS

In order to promote good wound healing, smoking should be stopped for several weeks before and after surgery. Studies show that people who continue to smoke after endoscopic sinus surgery do not have as successful an outcome. Smoking causes more post-surgical problems—most commonly, a need for further surgery—than allergies, asthma, or prior surgeries.

Possible Complications

FESS is a safe and minimally invasive procedure, and complications are rare. Still, any surgery carries some degree of risk. Bleeding is the most common complication. If you experience extensive bleeding and swelling directly after the procedure, your physician will keep you overnight in the hospital. Infection is always a risk after surgery, but your doctor may prescribe antibiotics both before and after the procedure to help prevent this.

"EMPTY NOSE SYNDROME"

Some doctors believe that the surgical removal of too much turbinate tissue can result in "empty nose syndrome," an illness characterized by facial pain, crusting in the nose, breathing problems, bleeding, and depression. However, other physicians do not think this syndrome exists and attribute symptoms to causes such as poor surgical technique, a lack of good follow-up care, or other underlying medical problems. Only time and rigorous scientific study will determine who is right.

More-serious possible complications are septal perforation (a hole in the bone and cartilage separating the two sides of your nose), a diminished or lost sense of smell, vision problems including blindness, a cerebrospinal fluid leak, brain abscess, and meningitis. Post-surgical scarring and adhesions can lead to further obstruction and hence more sinus problems down the line. If you experience any unusual symptoms following surgery, see your doctor.

WHEN MORE EXTENSIVE SURGERY IS NECESSARY

At times more extensive surgery is necessary. For example, chronic invasive fungal sinusitis requires an open, external approach along with a full course of antifungal therapy. In serious cases like this, surgeons remove all affected soft tissue and bone. Extreme care must be taken in these circumstances not to tear sensitive surrounding structures such as the dura or orbital periosteum.

DENTAL SURGERY

When a person has stubborn, treatment-resistant maxillary sinusitis, sometimes doctors find that an infected tooth lies at the root of the problem. For example, there may be an upper tooth that has an irritating filling material, or perhaps an embedded, infected tooth root was left behind following an extraction. In cases like these, your doctor will refer you to a dentist for evaluation and possible surgical removal of the problem tooth.

COPING WITH SERIOUS COMPLICATIONS

The two most serious complications of sinusitis are orbital (eye) and intracranial (brain). Due to the wide availability of antibiotics in this country, today such severe complications occur much less frequently than they did in the past. Yet even in our modern antibiotic era, three out of four eye infections are due to sinus disease, and 10 percent of these result in visual loss. The key to reducing the severity of complications is early diagnosis and aggressive treatment, which often entails surgical intervention.

Orbital (Eye) Complications

Among the most frequent complications of sinusitis are those that involve the orbits—the two sockets that contain the eyeball and associated blood vessels, muscles, and nerves. Orbital complications are most often seen in children, although they can occur at any age. Their severity and the consequent need for surgery increases as you grow older. If the eyeball or optic nerve is affected, orbital inflammation can lead to a temporary or permanent loss of vision.

THE WARNING SIGNS OF EYE COMPLICATIONS

- Redness and swelling of the skin around the eye
- A swollen eyelid that bulges or protrudes
- Limited ability to move the eye (ophthalmoplegia)
- A protruding or bulging eyeball (proptosis)
- Drooping of the upper eyelid (ptosis)
- Swelling of the conjunctiva, the transparent mucous membrane covering the white of the eye and lining the inside of the eyelids (chemosis)
- An abnormal sensitivity to light (photophobia)
- Eye pain
- Double vision
- Blurred vision
- Fever
- Elevated white blood cell count

The Orbits and the Sinuses

Anatomically speaking, the orbits of the eyes are very closely linked with the sinuses. The frontals lie above the orbits in the forehead area, just below them in the cheekbones are the maxillaries, and to either side are the ethmoid and sphenoid sinuses. Ethmoid sinusitis is most commonly implicated in orbital complications, followed in order by maxillary and frontal infection. The sphenoids are only rarely involved.

Of course, in normal, healthy sinuses, this close proximity is not a cause for concern. Indeed, even when problems occur, the bony walls of the sinuses act as a natural deterrent to the spread of infection. But in some cases, protective mechanisms fail due to circumstances such as congenital malformations, tumors, recent or old fractures, surgical procedures, or infiltration by destructive bacteria or fungi. There are two ways in which sinus infection can extend into the orbits:

- Directly through the sinuses' bony walls, through congenital malformations, foramina (small openings in bone through which nerves pass), or erosion of the bony barrier.
- Through the network of veins that offers a free form of communication between the sinus cavities and orbits—these veins may contain infected thrombi, or clots. (This is known as retrograde thrombophlebitis.)

Why Orbital Complications Develop

Prior to the advent of antibiotics, complications from sinusitis were extremely common. In those years, as many as two in ten people who experienced orbital complications became blind as a result, and nearly that number developed meningitis (a potentially life-threatening inflammation of the meninges, the three membranes that enclose and protect the brain and spinal cord). With the wide availability of antibiotics, these figures have decreased. Today orbital complications are apt to occur for the following reasons:

- Impaired immunity
- Infection with a particularly virulent or drug-resistant microorganism
- Inadequate medical treatment
- A delay in surgical intervention

The Progression of Orbital Complications

There are six categories of orbital complications. Prompt medical attention is required in each case, for if eye problems are not aggressively treated, they become progressively more severe. The complications are listed below:

- *Periorbital or preseptal cellulitis* is the most common orbital complication, accounting for more than eight out of ten cases. Also known as inflammatory edema, this is an abnormal infectious swelling in the eyelid. Symptoms include redness and inflammation around the eye, and a swollen, protruding eyelid. In this condition, there is no limitation of eye movement and no impairment of visual acuity.

- In *orbital cellulitis,* infection extends beyond the eyelid into the soft tissue of the orbit. There may be varying degrees of paralysis of the eye muscles (ophthalmoplegia) and protrusion or bulging of the eyeball (proptosis). If the veins of the eye become blocked, conjunctival problems can develop. These include chemosis, or swelling of the conjunctiva (the transparent mucous membrane covering the white of the eye and lining the inside of the eyelids). There may also be decreased visual acuity. Left untreated, cellulitis can progress to abscess and blindness.

- A *subperiosteal abscess* is a collection of pus between the bony wall of the orbit and the periosteum of the orbit. Also called the periorbita, the periosteum is a tough, fibrous membrane covering the orbital contents. In the early stages of this condition, eye movement and vision generally remain intact. But as the infection advances, both deteriorate, and the abscess may penetrate into the orbit or eyelid. Chemosis (swelling of the conjunctiva) also develops.

- An *orbital abscess* is a collection of pus in the orbital tissue. It may occur as a spread of infection from subperiosteal abscess or as a complication of orbital cellulitis. Common consequences include conjunctival swelling (chemosis), paralysis of the eye muscles (ophthalmoplegia), protrusion or bulging of the eyeball (proptosis), and loss of vision.

- *Orbital apex syndrome* is a complication of sphenoid or posterior ethmoidal sinusitis. This condition affects the cranial nerves that pass through or near the sinuses. Although there is no significant inflammation or bulging of the eyeball (proptosis), further examination reveals neuropathy of multiple cranial nerves and possibly loss of vision. Orbital apex syndrome may be caused by fungal or bacterial infection. Other names for this complication are sphenoidal-ocular syndrome, superior orbital (sphenoidal) syndrome, and posterior orbital cellulitis.

- *Cavernous sinus thrombosis (CST),* the most severe form of orbital complication, is a potentially life-threatening condition. [Read more about CST beginning on the next page, under "Intracranial (Brain) Complications."]

Surgery for Orbital Complications
Surgeons commonly treat eye complications and underlying sinusitis at the same time. For example, during the same procedure, they drain both the orbital abscess and any involved sinuses. Sometimes surgery is external, but more often doctors perform FESS. Physicians recom-

---

THE CAUSES OF VISION IMPAIRMENT

- Damage to the optic nerve and retina through compression of the eye's circulation (ischemic neuropathy)
- Direct pressure on the optic nerve (compressive neuropathy)
- Reaction of the optic nerve to nearby infection (inflammatory optic neuropathy)

---

mend surgical intervention for orbital complications under the following circumstances:

- When there is an abscess
- When vision loss is severe
- If the disease has progressed for more than twenty-four hours
- If there is no sign of improvement after forty-eight to seventy-two hours of treatment with antibiotics

Intracranial (Brain) Complications

Serious brain infections can develop as a complication either of acute sinusitis or of a flare-up of chronic disease. For reasons that are not entirely clear, they occur most frequently in adolescent boys. Frontal sinusitis is the number one cause, followed by infections of the ethmoid, sphenoid, and maxillary sinuses. In one study, one out of ten people who were hospitalized for frontal sinusitis developed intracranial complications. The sinus infection can spread through infected bone, by way of infected veins that communicate with the brain, or through anatomic defects between the sinuses and the brain. Brain complications are life-threatening. They may progress to delirium, convulsions, coma, and death.

Types of Brain Complications

While meningitis is probably the one with which people are most familiar, intracranial complications take a number of different forms, including:

- *Osteitis and Osteomyelitis* Spread of infection into the bone is known as osteitis. Osteitis can be a serious complication of sinusitis that requires intensive antibiotic therapy and sometimes surgery. Left untreated, osteitis can progress to osteomyelitis, an even more severe infection of the bones and bone marrow. This typically causes erosion of the frontal bone (the bone at the front of the skull that forms the forehead and the roots of the eye sockets) and leads to a pus-filled swelling in the forehead called Pott's puffy tumor. Fortunately, with the wide availability of antibiotics today, osteomyelitis is increasingly rare.

▪ *Epidural Abscess* Osteitis can also lead to a collection of pus between the dura (a protective membrane surrounding the brain) and the inner surface of the skull. Symptoms are generally subtle and include increasing headache and low-grade fever.

▪ *Subdural Empyema* A subdural empyema can occur by direct spread from an epidural abscess, or from retrograde thrombophlebitis (the passage of infected clots through infected veins). The subdural space lies between the dura and the arachnoid, the outermost and the middle of the three membranes that cover and protect the skull. A subdural empyema is a collection of pus in the subdural space. As this condition progresses over the cerebral hemispheres, it causes further swelling and increased intracranial pressure. Early symptoms of subdural empyema include headache and fever, which are followed by partial or complete paralysis of one side of the body, facial nerve paralysis, and seizures. In the late stages of the infection, there is nausea, vomiting, a slowed heart rate, and hypertension. Death may result.

▪ *Brain Abscess* Brain abscesses most frequently occur as a complication of frontal sinusitis and usually affect the frontal lobe of the brain. This is the largest part of the cerebrum and one that plays a significant role in personality and mental processes. When the abscess develops slowly, symptoms are subtle and may include only slight changes in mood or behavior. With brain swelling, intracranial pressure increases. If the abscess ruptures into the ventricles, death quickly occurs.

▪ *Meningitis* Meningitis is an inflammation of the meninges, the membranes that cover the brain and spinal cord. Unlike other intracranial complications, this disease is rarely due to frontal sinusitis alone. More commonly, it is linked with an extension of ethmoid or sphenoid infection. The symptoms of meningitis may include a severe headache, fever, seizures, and irritability. Infection may progress to delirium, drowsiness, seizures, coma, and death.

▪ *Cavernous Sinus Thrombosis* As we mentioned earlier, cavernous sinus thrombosis (CST) can develop as a result of orbital complications. Alternatively, infection of the cavernous sinuses—two large blood reservoirs that lie on either side of the sphenoids—may occur as a direct extension of ethmoid or sphenoid sinusitis, or as a result of epidural or subdural abscesses. Its early symptoms include fever, headache, abnormal sensitivity to light (photophobia), double vision, and swollen eyelids. These signs may soon be joined by drooping of the upper eyelid (ptosis), a bulging eye (proptosis), conjunctival swelling (chemosis), paralysis of the eye muscles (ophthalmoplegia), and loss of vision. Your doctor can confirm a diagnosis of CST if symptoms affect both eyes, which other orbital complications normally do not do. A further spread of infection can lead to meningitis, cerebral thrombosis (potentially fatal blood clots in the brain), and abscesses.

▪ *Superior Sagittal Sinus Thrombosis* This life-threatening condition is caused by retrograde thrombophlebitis from frontal sinusitis. Superior sagittal sinus thrombosis (SSST) often occurs along with epidural, subdural, or brain abscesses. Its symptoms include nausea, vomiting, and a severe headache. Depending upon the location of the clot, other problems may also develop. These range from motor and sensory deficits and changes in mental status, all the way to seizures and coma. Even with antibiotic therapy, this disease proves fatal in nearly eight out of ten people.

Surgery for Brain Complications

As with eye surgery, in order to decrease the need for future surgery and prevent any further spread of infection, whenever possible an intracranial (brain) complication and underlying sinusitis are treated in a single, combined procedure. Extensive surgery has proven more effective than limited procedures in decreasing the need for future surgery. However, if this is not possible, the immediate goal is to drain infected fluid trapped within the sinuses and brain. Later procedures will involve altering sinus anatomy to improve drainage and thus prevent future infection.

The treatment of brain abscesses depends on their location and the patient's condition. Aspiration (removal by suction) and excision (surgically cutting off diseased tissue) are the two methods used. A craniotomy is a type of incision in which the surgeon opens a part of the skull to drain fluid. However, in recent years, aspiration has been the procedure of choice. When it is possible, aspiration is a less extensive and traumatic procedure than excision, and there are fewer recurrences of infection. When osteomyelitis leads to wide infection and erosion of the frontal bone, debridement—the surgical removal of damaged or infected tissue to expose the healthy tissue beneath—is required.

MAINTAIN REALISTIC EXPECTATIONS

To recap, surgery should be considered only when all other treatment avenues have been exhausted. If you and your doctor do decide that surgery is your best option, dramatic technological advances make the experience far less traumatic than it was only two short decades ago. And in certain circumstances—such as serious complications— surgery is a must. But do keep in mind that it is not a sure cure for the pain and inflammation of chronic sinusitis and that people with relatively mild disease or specific localized problems tend to fare best. Most important, before you make a final decision, carefully explore all the possible risks and benefits of surgery with your doctor.

CHAPTER 8
_____

Sinus Problems in Children

It is especially important to control sinus disease in children. In addition to relieving their current discomfort, preventing chronic or recurrent infections during childhood can offer protection from sinus problems later in life. Otherwise, childhood disease can lead to life-long difficulties with sinusitis due to scar tissue formation that interferes with normal drainage.

CHILDREN ARE ESPECIALLY SUSCEPTIBLE

While a runny nose is most commonly a sign of a cold, persistent congestion in a child can also be a symptom of sinusitis. For a number of reasons, children are particularly susceptible to this disease. First of all, their sinuses have yet to fully develop and thus are physically smaller than those of adults. This means that a relatively minor amount of swelling can lead to more significant obstruction than in older individuals. Also, children have immature immune systems, a circumstance that makes them prone to frequent infections. In fact, children average anywhere from three to eight colds or upper respiratory viruses a year, which can lead to acute sinusitis (which lasts four weeks or less) or even to more persistent, chronic problems. Furthermore, environmental influences play a prominent role in pediatric sinus infection. Children in day care are routinely exposed to viruses and are more likely than children in home care to experience prolonged respiratory symptoms. Exposure to environmental tobacco smoke also takes a special toll on young, developing lungs, and children who live in a damp house with parents who smoke face a doubled risk of rhinitis. Then too, problems with adenoids or reflux may contribute to sinus disease.

CHILDREN ARE NOT JUST MINIATURE ADULTS

Of course, these are far from the only differences between sinusitis in children and in adults. Symptoms are usually subtler in youngsters. It is easy for parents (and even doctors) to attribute the persistent runny noses and coughs of sinusitis to a cold or allergy. This means that affected children are undertreated. On the other hand, many are also overtreated. Since it is more challenging to differentiate a viral upper respiratory infection (URI) from sinusitis in children than in adults, physicians sometimes mistakenly prescribe antibiotics for children with colds.

Further complicating diagnosis is the fact that small children can't articulate what is wrong with them. And because children are not simply small adults, treatment differs. For example, the surgical techniques applied to adults are usually not appropriate—and can even prove harmful—for youngsters. Except in cases of complicated sinusitis or chronic disease that fails to respond to all other possible treatments, otolaryngologists—specialists in sinus disease—generally do not recommend functional endoscopic sinus surgery (FESS) for children.

THE ANATOMY OF CHILDREN'S SINUSES

To briefly review sinus anatomy: Four pairs of sinuses are connected to the nasal cavity by small openings called ostia. Small maxillary (behind the cheek) and ethmoid (between the eyes) sinuses are present at birth. The maxillaries enlarge rapidly until age three and once more between ages seven and twelve, until they are fully developed in adulthood. These sinuses play a particularly large part in childhood sinusitis and are often slightly larger in males. Behind the maxillary sinuses and between the bony orbits are the ethmoids, which are almost fully developed by the age of twelve. There are two types of ethmoid sinuses: anterior and posterior. Because they are so close to the eyes, the ethmoids are the sinuses most frequently implicated in eye-related complications, which are especially common in children.

The frontal sinuses in the forehead are very tiny at birth but are fairly developed by age twelve. Frontal sinusitis is the primary cause of intracranial, or brain, complications, which occur most frequently in adolescent boys. While young children who develop acute sinusitis usually respond well to antibiotics, adolescents—for reasons that remain unknown—often don't and as a result go on to develop complications. Sometimes one of the frontal sinuses is congenitally underdeveloped or missing altogether. The sphenoid sinuses are located deeper in the skull in the upper region of the nose and behind the eyes. These sinuses, which are not present at birth, begin to develop around age three and are extensively developed by age seven.

WHAT CAUSES SINUSITIS IN CHILDREN?

Even though it takes some years for the sinuses to fully develop, this does not mean that children cannot get sinus infections. As with adults, anything that causes swelling in the nose—such as inflammation associated with a cold or allergic reaction—can have a negative impact on a child's sinuses. Sinus disease in youngsters may develop due to the closing off of ostia; the malfunction of cilia, small hairs that normally propel the mucous blanket through the sinuses; or a change in the amount or consistency of mucus.

As with adults, acute sinusitis in children is most commonly associated with upper respiratory viruses. Similarly, too, there is usually no one single cause of disease. For example, a child who is in day care is apt to experience more frequent and persistent colds, which can lead to sinusitis. If that same child has allergies, he or she is even more susceptible. Other contributing factors include environmental influences, allergies, adenoid problems, reflux, immunodeficiency, congenital abnormalities, and diseases such as cystic fibrosis. Although, for a long time, experts believed that anatomic variations around the osteomeatal unit—such as deviated septums or concha bullosae—were associated with chronic sinusitis in children, recent studies do not show this to be the case. Sometimes parents are surprised to find that the cause of symptoms is a small foreign body such as a raisin, peanut, or bead lodged inside a youngster's nose.

Upper Respiratory Infections

Acute sinusitis is most often preceded by a common cold, which is caused by a virus. Most cases of sinus disease occur in the winter, when upper respiratory infections are at their peak. These viruses cause inflammation and swelling that block the sinus ostia. Mucus that normally drains into the nasal passages is instead trapped in the sinuses, making them a fertile breeding ground for bacteria and fungi.

As mentioned earlier, differentiating sinusitis from a URI is especially challenging in children. It is difficult even for a pediatrician to determine the point at which a primary cold ends and a secondary, bacterial infection takes over. Invasive testing called aspiration is the only sure way to confirm the diagnosis—and the procedure is both unnecessary and undesirable in most cases. In adults, cold symptoms that persist for longer than ten days are a sign that sinusitis may be the problem. Yet even this guideline does not always hold true for children. While the average duration of a viral URI is less than ten days in children, upper respiratory tract symptoms may persist. For example, congestion and a runny nose may linger for longer than fifteen days in more than one in ten toddlers in day care. Contrary to popular opinion, a change in the color or texture of nasal discharge is also not a specific symptom of bacterial infection.

So what is a parent to do? Even though they are not certain signs of sinusitis, your index of suspicion should be raised when your child experiences a viral URI that is no better after ten days or that worsens after five to seven days. Possible symptoms include congestion, nasal discharge, postnasal drip, facial pressure or pain (especially when located around one sinus), ear pressure or pain, a reduced sense of smell, fever, cough, fatigue, and maxillary dental pain. Bring your child to the pediatrician for evaluation and treatment. If the problem continues, ask for a referral to an otolaryngologist, who is specially trained in the diagnosis and treatment of sinus disease. Your doctor will prescribe drugs such as antibiotics to cure the infection. In the meantime, keep your child as comfortable as possible with simple home-care measures, such as getting adequate rest, drinking clear fluids, using a humidifier, and taking over-the-counter medication such as Tylenol to relieve discomfort. (Remember that aspirin is not recommended for children or adolescents because of the risk of Reye's syndrome.)

Environmental Factors

Researchers have discovered that children with chronic sinusitis often have one of two primary environmental influences in common: they are in day care or are frequently exposed to environmental tobacco smoke. Although often an essential part of family life, day care centers are hotbeds of infection, especially for very young children with immature immune systems. On the other hand, their impact pales when compared with dangerous exposure to secondhand smoke, which puts children at risk not only for sinusitis but also for lung problems such as asthma. Older children put themselves at significant additional risk if they smoke themselves or abuse recreational drugs such as inhalants. As with adults, pollutants in the environment also contribute to sinusitis in children. Fortunately, there are many steps that you as a parent can take to protect your child from risky environmental influences.

Choose a Safe Day-Care Facility

Infectious microorganisms are particularly prevalent in day-care settings, and more frequent exposure to ill contacts has long been known to increase the risk and protract the length of acute sinusitis. To reduce your child's exposure to germs, your best bet is to look for the cleanest possible facility, and one with a small number of children. Make sure that frequent hand washing is a rule; this simple measure goes a long way to thwart the spread of infection. Whether or not your infant is in day care, you can help strengthen his or her immune system through breastfeeding, as studies show that breastfed children have fewer colds.

Limit Exposure to Environmental Tobacco Smoke

Passive smoking is associated with a variety of health problems in children. Environmental tobacco smoke is a potent trigger of respiratory symptoms, from coughing and wheezing to asthma attacks. Children who are exposed to secondhand smoke also experience an increased risk of rhinitis, sinusitis, and allergic sensitization (probably due to the fact that the production of IgE antibodies is enhanced by cigarette smoking).

When it comes to secondhand smoke, put your foot down: there is no reason for your child to be exposed to this unnecessary health risk. While it is difficult to get smokers to quit, simply making them aware of the dangers secondhand smoke poses to children is a powerful incentive. However, if a family member or close friend can't or won't quit, at least make certain that no one smokes in the presence of your child. In particular, discourage smoking at any time in confined spaces such as the home or car.

Allergies

Swollen mucous membranes due to allergies may also lead to ostial obstruction and consequent sinusitis. But perhaps because their symptoms are so similar and often overlap, there is much confusion regarding the relationship between allergies and pediatric sinusitis. There appears to be a close connection: eight out of ten children with chronic sinusitis have allergic disorders. However, episodes of sinusitis are most common in the winter months, when viral upper respiratory infections—*not* seasonal allergies—are at their peak. Thus it may be that in pediatric sinusitis, environmental and food allergies play a greater role than seasonal allergies.

Controlling Allergies

The bottom line is that if allergies are an underlying problem, it is essential to control them in order to control sinusitis. Otherwise, inflammation caused by allergic reactions can lead to bout after bout of sinus infection. Especially if there is a family history, keep a lookout for allergic symptoms in your child. Common signs include congestion, stuffiness, nasal discharge, an itchy nose, sneezing, and cough. Younger children who have allergies may demonstrate behavioral changes, while older ones can have headaches that may be accompanied by facial pressure or pain. Other indications are the "allergic shiner" (in which there is a puffy, bluish discoloration of the lower eyelids) and the "allergic salute" (a common gesture in allergic children, in which the nose is wiped vertically with the palm). Clues in infants are colic, poor sleeping habits, irritability, and frequent formula changes necessitated by diarrhea or vomiting.

To control allergies, it is important to identify and eliminate suspected allergens from your child's environment. Commonly inhaled allergens that are present year-round include house dust mites, animal dander, and molds. As they are exposed in successive seasons to tree, grass, and weed pollens, children may also develop seasonal allergies. Common food allergens include dairy products, soybeans, wheat, corn, eggs, and peanuts. Some children outgrow food sensitivity, but many do not. As with middle-ear infections (or otitis media, with which sinusitis shares many similarities), eliminating items such as dairy products from the diet improves symptoms. But in some cases, additional treatment—such as medication or immunotherapy (allergy shots)—is required.

Adenoids

When enlarged or infected, these clusters of tissue at the back of the nose and throat may also contribute to sinus disease. Although an exact cause-and-effect relationship has yet to be established, adenoids are thought to factor into sinusitis in one of two ways. If they are infected, the infection can spread to the sinuses; if they are very large, they cause stasis of secretions (stoppage of normal flow) and obstruction, which can result in infection. Some children outgrow this condition, while others require surgery.

Cleft Palate

Children born with a gap in the roof of the mouth are apt to have problems with breathing, eating, and speaking. Sinusitis is a common complication of a cleft palate. Potential medical explanations for this association are an incompetent velopharynx, a deviated nasal septum, an underdeveloped maxillary sinus, and impaired mucociliary function. In simpler terms, when there is no palate separating the mouth and nose, there is possible contamination and irritation of delicate mucous membranes every time a child eats and drinks. This sets the stage for infection. Cleft palates require surgical correction, which is usually accomplished before the age of two.

Cystic Fibrosis

Characterized by persistent lung infections, cystic fibrosis (CF) is a genetic disorder that causes abnormally thickened mucus. This often leads to blockage of the sinus ostia and consequent infection. Children with this disease are especially prone to chronic sinusitis, which as usual is treated with antibiotics, nasal steroids, and nasal irrigation. Surgery may be necessary to correct problems such as persistent nasal obstruction; studies have shown pediatric functional endoscopic sinus surgery (FESS) to be a safe and effective option for youngsters with CF. In recent years, there have been significant advances in the treatment of cystic fibrosis. As a result, affected children are living longer and experiencing a higher quality of life. An especially promising new area of research for future treatment lies in gene therapy.

Gastroesophageal Reflux Disease

In recent years, there has been a greater understanding of the relationship between gastroesophageal reflux disease (GERD) and chronic sinusitis in children. Reflux is characterized by the backward flow of acid from the stomach up into the esophagus. When reflux penetrates into the pharynx and nose, nasal tissues become irritated and swollen and there may be impaired mucociliary clearance. If the sinus ostia are obstructed, infection can result. While adults experience obvious symptoms of GERD such as heartburn and regurgitation, this disease affects children more subtly and insidiously. For this reason, reflux in children is sometimes referred to as silent GERD. Treatment consists of behavioral and dietary modifications, acid-reducing and pro-kinetic medications, and possibly surgery. Good reflux management can greatly reduce the need for surgery in children with chronic sinusitis.

Immunodeficiency

Immunodeficiency is also associated with chronic sinusitis in children. Like adults, children with weakened immune systems are more susceptible to infections of all kinds, including chronic sinusitis. Immunodeficiency is associated with a number of different causes, including chemotherapy, bone marrow transplants, and HIV infection. Problems that are rarely seen in healthy children—such as fungal sinusitis—occasionally occur in youngsters with compromised immune systems. Children with immunodeficiency may require intravenous gamma globulin therapy. Interestingly, studies show that children with repeated viral infections at an early age are less likely to develop asthma; this research supports the theory that repeated viral infections (with the exception of lower respiratory infections) stimulate the immune systems of young children into the type that is less likely to develop atopic allergy.

Other Causes of Sinusitis

Sinusitis in children also has a variety of other causes. Scars from prior surgery, fractures, or infection may contribute to chronic sinusitis, while foreign bodies (such as small buttons or toys) occasionally find their way into juvenile noses and cause problems. Other systemic diseases can also play a role in sinusitis. For example, primary ciliary dyskinesia is a rare disorder in which tiny hairs called cilia fail to sweep mucus out of the sinuses, resulting in poor mucous drainage and consequent infection. Sinus disease may also be associated with congenital abnormalities such as a significantly deviated nasal septum or concha bullosa, although these are currently believed to play a lesser role than thought in the past. Nevertheless, structural defects like these can cause alterations in sinus development and drainage.

DOES ASTHMA PLAY A ROLE IN SINUSITIS?

At least half of those treated for asthma also have nasal or sinus symptoms. It is clear that sinusitis and nasal polyp disease make asthma worse; however, there is no clear evidence that asthma makes sinusitis worse.

SINUSITIS SYMPTOMS

As with adults, cold symptoms that persist for ten days or longer are the most common signs of acute sinusitis. The symptoms themselves vary widely from child to child, and even from one age to the next. Younger children are most likely to have a persistent runny nose, while older children are more apt to experience postnasal drip. This may in turn lead to a sore throat, bad breath, nausea, or vomiting. At times, congestion can become so severe that a child cannot breathe through his or her nose. In some cases, the sense of smell diminishes or disappears altogether.

Coughing is another common symptom. A youngster may cough both day and night, although the problem is typically worse at night. Children who suffer from both sinusitis and asthma may find themselves racked by particularly troublesome coughing fits, and asthma attacks can be aggravated by sinusitis.

Sinus disease can also be painful. Because children who are not verbal express this in a number of different ways, be on the alert for signs such as unusual irritability or head banging. The location of sinus pain depends on which sinus is affected. For example, infection in the maxillary sinuses causes facial pressure or pain that mimics a toothache, while ethmoid inflammation may lead to pain between the eyes. Children over the age of six may also experience headaches, especially upon waking in the morning.

Symptoms Can Be Subtle

The symptoms of sinusitis are often difficult to recognize. Parents may not even realize that a child has acute sinusitis when it occurs secondary to a cold and clears up on its own without treatment. And while acute sinusitis may masquerade as a cold, the signs of chronic sinusitis are even more subtle and easy to overlook. These symptoms last longer than four weeks, and may continue for months or even years. They include headaches, pain around the eyes and cheeks, tenderness of the sinuses to pressure and touch, fever, and difficulty breathing through the nose. While adults experience fatigue and a general feeling of illness or malaise, children with chronic sinusitis are more likely to be cranky and irritable. It is important not to disregard these signs, for left untreated, sinusitis can lead to serious complications.

MAKING THE DIAGNOSIS

If you suspect that your child has sinusitis, see your pediatrician for proper diagnosis and treatment. Doctors diagnose sinus infection through a description of symptoms, physical examination, and various tests. Be sure to tell the physician if your child has allergies or has recently had a cold, as these factors may contribute to acute sinusitis.

Physical Examination

During examination, physicians use a technique called percussion— gently tapping with the fingers—to detect any tenderness in the sinus areas. This is a sign of infection. If you consult an otolaryngologist, he or she may examine your child's nasal passages using a long, lighted tube called an endoscope. This instrument is inserted into a

---

COMMON SYMPTOMS OF SINUSITIS IN CHILDREN

- A "cold" that lasts for longer than ten days
- Purulent nasal discharge
- Postnasal drip
- A cough that may be more severe at night
- Nasal airway obstruction
- Irritability or fatigue
- Swelling around the eyes
- Fever
- Headache (usually after age six)

---

nostril and threaded into the nasal passages. Endoscopy reveals unusual narrowing or obstruction, inflammation, swelling, structural deformities, secretions, and polyps. Polyps are unusual growths in children, but sometimes occur in cases of cystic fibrosis or allergic fungal sinusitis.

Of course, physical examination of a child (especially if it includes endoscopy) can be quite a challenge. Not surprisingly, unhappy infants and toddlers squirm, move their heads from side to side, and cry. Even older children may balk at the idea. Because abrupt movements and tears obstruct examination, parents can help by soothing their children and keeping them calm. Prior to endoscopy, the doctor will use an anesthetic spray or liquid to make insertion less uncomfortable.

Tests for Sinusitis

When sinusitis is not clinically obvious or when chronic infection is suspected, further testing may be necessary. In recent years, CT scanning has emerged as the best technique for diagnosing chronic sinusitis in children. MRI (magnetic resonance imaging) is used less often. This technique is primarily useful in diagnosing eye and brain complications, and it takes longer than CT to perform—thus many children cannot tolerate MRI without sedation. X rays are not particularly beneficial, since they tend to either overstate or understate the nature of disease.

Another helpful test is a culture of sinus drainage. This can identify the microorganism that is responsible for the infection. Other possible tests include sweat chloride tests (for cystic fibrosis), ciliary function tests, HIV tests, tests for immunodeficiency, and allergy testing.

MEDICAL TREATMENT

As many as four in ten cases of acute sinusitis in children resolve on their own without treatment. However, chronic sinusitis is a more intractable disease, which invariably requires aggressive medical treatment. Since most sinus infections are caused by bacteria, antibiotics are the cornerstone of therapy.

Antibiotics

Types of antibiotics prescribed for sinusitis include the penicillin, cephalosporin, macrolide, and sulfa groups. In chronic or recurrent cases, the newer, broad-spectrum forms are recommended. Other considerations your physician will take into account include your child's overall health, allergies to any medications, possible side effects, cost, and convenience. Treatment varies according to the relative severity of the problem. Carefully follow your pediatrician's instructions regarding dosage, and make certain that your child takes the entire course of antibiotics prescribed (even if his or her symptoms disappear). (Turn to chapter 6 for a more comprehensive discussion of antibiotics and other medications for sinusitis.)

THE GOALS OF ANTIBIOTIC THERAPY

- To restore the sinuses to health
- To prevent the development of chronic sinus disease
- To avoid the development of serious complications such as meningitis or vision loss

---

Acute Sinusitis

Acute disease is usually treated for ten to fourteen days. If symptoms persist, antibiotics are given for twenty-one days. The first group of antibiotics below is preferable, because effectiveness of the second group against the major bacteria that cause acute sinusitis is limited—bacterial failure of 20 to 25 percent is possible. In addition, sulfa drugs (which include Bactrim, Cotrim, and Septra) have been associated with an increased risk of life-threatening toxic epidural necrolysis (also known as Stevens-Johnson syndrome, a condition characterized by severe eruptions around the mouth, eyes, or anus). When acute sinusitis is caused by *Streptococcus pneumoniae* bacteria, your doctor will probably prescribe Augmentin (amoxicillin-clavulanate). If Augmentin proves ineffective, Cleocin (clindamycin)—a drug that has more potential GI side effects—is also a good alternative.

The four drugs below are the initial ones prescribed for children with acute disease:

- Amoxicillin (Amoxil and Trimox) is one of the most frequently prescribed drugs for children—it is inexpensive, tastes good (like pink bubblegum), and effective. Because it is a penicillin antibiotic, children who are allergic to penicillin should *not* take this drug.
- Amoxicillin-clavulanate (Augmentin) combines amoxicillin with clavulanic acid to "augment" its effectiveness. To avoid intestinal irritation, give Augmentin to your child with food or milk. Because it is a penicillin antibiotic, children who are allergic to penicillin should *not* take this drug.
- Cefpodoxime proxetil (Vantin) is a cephalosporin antibiotic. A small percentage of people who are allergic to penicillin are also allergic to cephalosporins.
- Cefuroxime axetil (Ceftin) is also a cephalosporin antibiotic. Taking cephalosporins with food or milk can help prevent stomach upset.

If your child is allergic to the above drugs, which are known as beta-lactams, one of the following medications will be recommended:

- Azithromycin (Zithromax) is an unusual antibiotic in that it is taken only once a day for five days. It is important to take Zithromax on an empty stomach.
- Clarithromycin (Biaxin), like Zithromax, is a macrolide antibiotic. Zithromax and Biaxin should not be given to children who are allergic to erythromycin.
- Erythromycin (E.E.S., E-Mycin, ERYC, EryPed, Ery-Tab, Erythrocin, Ilosone, PCE, and Pediamycin) is a good alternative for children who are sensitive or allergic to penicillin antibiotics. It is one of the safest antibiotics available today.
- Trimethoprim-sulfamethoxazole (Bactrim, Cotrim, and Septra) is a combination drug that is more powerful than either of its individual components. Sulfamethoxazole is a sulfonamide or sulfa drug—these have been associated with rare but potentially

fatal reactions such as toxic epidural necrolysis (Stevens-Johnson syndrome). Sulfa drugs also cause heightened light sensitivity and interact with many other medications.

COMMON BACTERIA IN CHILDHOOD SINUSITIS

Seven out of ten acute or recurrent childhood infections are caused by the following three bacteria:

- *Streptococcus pneumoniae*
- *Moraxella catarrhalis*
- *Hemophilus influenzae*

Special Considerations in Children

When it comes to medications and children, certain special considerations must be taken into account. Recommended doses of drugs are based on your child's weight as well as age; carefully follow your pediatrician's instructions regarding dosage. Children's reactions to medication are highly individual—even siblings can have very different reactions. If your child develops a troubling response to any drug, immediately discontinue it and call the pediatrician. Certain antibiotics called fluoroquinolones—gatifloxacin (Tequin), levofloxacin (Levaquin), and moxifloxacin (Avelox)—are not approved for use in children.

Switch Therapy

If your child's symptoms are unchanged or worsen after three days of antibiotic therapy, consult your pediatrician. He or she will want to reevaluate the youngster's condition, often by taking a culture of sinus drainage and switching to a different antibiotic. Possible choices include amoxicillin (Amoxil and Trimox), amoxicillin-clavulanate (Augmentin), cefpodoxime proxetil (Vantin), and cefuroxime axetil (Ceftin). Your pediatrician may also prescribe combination therapy with more than one antibiotic, even if your child has already been given antibiotics in the past six weeks. Combination therapy might include amoxicillin (Amoxil and Trimox) or clindamycin (Cleocin) with cefixime (Suprax) or cefpodoxime proxetil (Vantin) or trimethoprim-sulfamethoxazole (Bactrim, Cotrim, and Septra).

Side Effects and Adverse Reactions

Before giving any medication to your child, always ask your pediatrician about possible side effects and adverse reactions. The most common side effects of antibiotics are stomach upset and diarrhea. Giving your child medication after a meal may eliminate these problems. But the longer your child must take antibiotics, the more likely side effects are apt to occur. Taking antibiotics for longer than two weeks depletes the intestines of their normal intestinal flora, which can lead to diarrhea. Give your child yogurt with active cultures to restore normal intestinal balance. If he or she doesn't like or can't tolerate yogurt, ask your pediatrician about lactobacillus supplements.

In some cases, more severe adverse reactions occur. If your child develops reactions such as a fever or skin rash, discontinue medication and call the pediatrician. These can be signs of an allergic reaction. In rare cases, a severe and potentially life-threatening allergic reaction called anaphylaxis may occur. This is characterized by a sudden onset of hives, difficulty breathing, and an abrupt drop in blood pressure. Anaphylaxis is an emergency situation that demands immediate medical attention. In the future, your child should not be given that antibiotic or any other similar antibiotics.

GIVE YOUR CHILD ANTIBIOTICS EXACTLY AS YOUR DOCTOR PRESCRIBES

Whether your child has acute or chronic sinusitis, it is important to administer the entire course of medication just as the pediatrician instructs, even if the symptoms disappear before the medication runs out. Otherwise, the infection can return in a more virulent form, or your child may develop antibiotic resistance (or both).

Chronic Sinusitis

Chronic sinusitis is treated with a longer course of antibiotics than acute disease, on average four to six weeks. Therapy is with broad-spectrum antibiotics that cover the bacteria of acute sinusitis as well as *Staphylococcus aureus*. Initially, physicians recommend a two-week course of oral antibiotics. If symptoms do not improve in five to seven days, your doctor will switch drugs. If there is still no change for another five to seven days, a culture of sinus drainage should be analyzed and other causes of symptoms considered. When a child slowly responds to treatment, another two-week course is prescribed.

Prophylactic treatment—that is, preventive treatment with smaller-than-usual antibiotic dosages—may be helpful in some cases (for instance, in children with immune suppression due to chemotherapy). However, prophylactic therapy has come under increasing fire in recent years, due to its association with emerging resistant bacteria. As a result, physicians are very cautious in their use of this technique. Intravenous (IV) antibiotic therapy is another safe and effective alternative for resistant chronic cases and may be a reasonable alternative to functional endoscopic sinus surgery (FESS).

WHEN ANTIBIOTICS DON'T WORK

Children who do not respond to antibiotics require further evaluation, which may include CT scanning, fiberoptic endoscopy, or sinus aspiration with culture. Surgery is considered only when underlying causes such as passive smoke, reflux, and allergies have been controlled and systemic causes have been ruled out.

Beyond Antibiotics: Other Medications for Sinusitis

Many other medications are also recommended for sinusitis. For example, analgesic products containing acetaminophen (such as Tylenol) or ibuprofen (Advil or Motrin) can be given to children to control sinus pain. (Again, children and adolescents must never be given aspirin, which has been associated with a rare but life-threatening disorder called Reye's syndrome.) Topical decongestants are also helpful, but should not be used for more than three days. Otherwise, in a rebound effect, their regular use leads to even more congestion and swelling of nasal passages. Mucous thinners—such as plain Robitussin or other cold remedies that contain guaifenesin—are also beneficial. Some parents prefer Triaminic Expectorant, a decongestant-expectorant (guaifenesin) combination. Carefully follow the directions on the labels of all these over-the-counter medications.

Topical nasal steroid spray is another medication commonly prescribed to reduce the congestion and inflammation of acute or chronic sinusitis. These drugs are apt to be most effective in children who have chronic, nonpurulent sinusitis, with allergies as a strong contributing factor. Mometasone (Nasonex) is approved for children as young as two years old, and Flonase (fluticasone) is approved down to age four. However, doctors are still investigating the long-term safety risks of steroid sprays, especially in children. As a result, physicians carefully weigh their risks versus benefits and prescribe them with caution. If the decision is made to use steroid nasal sprays, nasal irrigation—cleansing the nose with a saltwater rinse—improves their effectiveness.

Nasal Irrigation

Rinsing the nose two to three times a day with a saltwater mixture washes away crusty debris, decongesting the nose, improving airflow, and making breathing easier. Salt water is one of the most effective ways to improve nasal hygiene. Because children may at first be fearful of nasal irrigation, it is best to ease them slowly into this process. Initiate irrigation in younger children with a pump spray container, such as one used for nasal steroid spray. Squirt several times into each side of the nose, while your child is in a sitting or standing position. In older children, use a bulb or ear syringe, a large (30 cc) medical syringe, or a water pick with an irrigation tap.

HOW TO MAKE A NASAL IRRIGATION RINSE

Commercial solutions are available, or you can make your own rinse:

- Fill a clean one-quart jar with tap or bottled water.
- Add two to three teaspoons of pickling or canning salt. Do not use table salt, which contains additives. If the mixture is too strong for your child, use less salt.
- Add one teaspoon of baking soda.
- Store at room temperature for up to one week, and stir or shake before each use.

Home Care for Sinusitis

Although home remedies are not a cure, the following tips may lessen the discomfort of sinusitis:

- Make sure your child drinks plenty of fluids in order to keep nasal discharge thin.
- Administer over-the-counter saline nasal spray to relieve discomfort.

- Apply gentle heat over tender, inflamed areas.
- Use a humidifier to increase delivery of moisture to the sinuses.
- Avoid temperature extremes, which can increase sinus pain.
- Inhale steam from a vaporizer to relieve sinus discomfort.
- Avoid exposure to environmental (secondhand) smoke and other pollutants.
- Carefully follow your physician's recommendations for the treatment of underlying conditions such as upper respiratory infections or allergies.

WHEN SURGERY IS NECESSARY

In children who experience serious complications, or in whom chronic sinusitis fails to respond to antibiotic therapy and optimal treatment of underlying conditions, surgery can be immensely beneficial. However, surgery is considered only when all other treatment options have been exhausted, or if there is a nasal obstruction that cannot be corrected with medication. In spite of dramatic technological advances, surgery on the narrow and fragile noses of children always involves some element of risk. Most recently, concern has focused on interference with sinus development and midfacial growth following endoscopic surgery in children. To reduce the element of risk, surgical procedures are performed by skilled specialists known as otolaryngologists.

Adenoidectomy

Before considering more extensive nasal surgery, doctors always check a child's adenoids. These masses of lymphoid tissue on the wall behind the nasal cavities provide a fertile breeding ground for bacteria and can cause stasis of nasal secretions. Adenoidectomy (the surgical removal of enlarged or infected adenoids) is a first-line treatment for stubborn chronic cases of pediatric sinusitis. Tonsillectomy and adenoidectomy, often done together and called T & A, were routinely performed until the 1970s. Today, however, it is recognized that the tonsils and adenoids help the body fight infection, and surgery takes place only if adenoids result in frequent bouts of sinusitis, strep throat, or middle-ear infections that do not respond to other treatments.

EYE COMPLICATIONS IN CHILDREN

Orbital, or eye, complications are most common in children. They can cause significant damage, including blindness, and in rare cases are even fatal. To control these dangerous complications, young children at risk are usually aggressively treated with intravenous antibiotics that cross the blood-brain barrier; older children more often require endoscopic drainage of abscesses. CT scanning is performed to diagnose eye complications.

Adenoidectomies are most frequently performed on children between the ages of one and seven. Surgery improves symptoms by eliminating stasis of secretions and by doing away with the adenoid pad as a potential location for bacterial colonization. The procedure takes place on an outpatient basis, with most children able to go home after several hours of observation. The most frequent complication is bleeding. Children who experience this problem should be placed on their sides, so they do not choke. In most cases, however, a sore throat is the only uncomfortable consequence. Plenty of liquids and soft food can help relieve the sore throat discomfort that may persist for up to two weeks following an adenoidectomy. Tylenol is the only recommended analgesic; do not give your child aspirin or ibuprofen, as these drugs have anticoagulant effects that can cause bleeding after surgery.

Functional Endoscopic Sinus Surgery (FESS)

In some cases, more extensive surgery is necessary. Not long ago, any sort of intranasal surgery in young children was considered complicated and dangerous. Indeed, otolaryngologists are still extremely cautious in their surgical recommendations for children. But with the advent of less invasive pediatric functional endoscopic sinus surgery (FESS), surgeons can now treat complications or resistant chronic disease in children more safely and effectively. FESS is less invasive

THE GOALS OF FESS

- To promote better sinus drainage and ventilation
- To remove as little tissue as possible
- To fix problems while preserving normal mucous membranes

than conventional surgery, complications are rare, and nine out of ten operations result in significant improvement. (For more information on FESS, turn to chapter 7.)

When FESS Is Recommended

FESS is performed in children for a variety of reasons. In some cases, it is necessary to clean and drain the sinuses. Other times, surgery is required to reopen or enlarge the natural openings of the sinuses to allow drainage. Absolute indications for surgery include brain or eye complications, fungal disease, polyps, and complete airway obstruction due to cystic fibrosis.

CT scanning is a useful guide when sinus surgery is necessary, but it should not be the sole determinant. This is because some studies have detected CT evidence of mucosal disease in as many as 50 percent of asymptomatic children under the age of twelve. As always, the goal is to avoid overtreatment as well as undertreatment of sinus disease.

Doctors view chronic sinusitis itself as only a relative indication for surgery. That is, surgery should be considered only when at least two to six weeks of antibiotic therapy has been exhausted, all accompanying diseases have been optimally treated, and any underlying systemic diseases have been ruled out.

INDICATIONS FOR ENDOSCOPIC SINUS SURGERY

- Complications of cystic fibrosis
- Antrochoanal polyps (these arise from the maxillary sinus and then protrude into the nose)
- Brain complications
- Mucoceles (swollen sacs or cavities filled with mucus) and mucopyceles (infected mucoceles)
- Orbital abscess (a collection of pus in the eye-socket tissue)
- Traumatic injury to the optic canal
- Dacrocystis (an inflammation of the tear sac that drains tears from the eye)
- Fungal sinusitis
- Some meningoencephaloceles (a herniation of brain and meningeal tissue through a defect in the brain's bony cover into an area outside the brain, such as the sinuses or nasal cavities and neoplasms (abnormal growths or tumors)

What to Expect

In young children, FESS is performed under general anesthesia. As they grow older, some youngsters are able to tolerate topical anesthesia. In the procedure, the surgeon uses a fiberoptic pediatric nasal endoscope for purposes such as enlarging a narrow sinus passage, or removing diseased tissue or a bone that is blocking a passage. This allows better drainage, making infection less likely. In some cases, powered instruments are employed to precisely remove growths ranging from small polyps to large tumors. Powered instrumentation reduces overall operating time and blood loss as compared with conventional methods. In problems such as cystic fibrosis, mucoceles, fungal sinusitis, and polyposis (multiple polyps), CT scanning is useful in determining the extent of surgery. Some surgeons pack the child's nose after surgery—however, the packs used are generally absorbable and do not require any subsequent removal.

After the Procedure

FESS is usually performed on an outpatient basis. However, if there are coexisting diseases such as asthma, or if a child experiences postoperative nausea and vomiting, to be on the safe side he or she will be kept overnight. At home, daily nasal saline irrigation is required. Your doctor will also prescribe two weeks of antibiotics, and intranasal steroid sprays for up to four months. Some children require a return to the operating room in two weeks for additional cleaning and draining of the sinuses under general anesthesia.

SINUSITIS AND CHILDREN

Sinusitis in children, while in many ways similar to that in adults, also has a number of significant differences. With their small nasal and sinus passages, even a little congestion can lead to a big problem in children. But the symptoms are usually subtle, making diagnosis a challenge. Treatment too is different—for example, doctors are even more conservative in recommending surgery in children than in adults. Perhaps most important, you can help protect children from developing sinusitis by limiting their exposure to toxic influences such as secondhand smoke and other environmental pollutants.

CHAPTER 9

Self-Care for Sinusitis

In an uncomplicated case of acute sinusitis, simple self-care measures are often all that is necessary to effect a cure. Even if you suffer from more serious chronic or recurrent acute disease, these same strategies can help you feel better and maybe even get well faster. Self-care measures are also beneficial in controlling health problems that are closely related to sinusitis, such as colds and allergies. Of course, maintaining a healthy lifestyle may prevent sinus disease from developing in the first place, or at least modify its severity and duration. Moreover, smart lifestyle choices are beneficial not only for your sinus health but also for your overall well-being.

SELF-CARE FOR THE SYMPTOMS OF SINUSITIS

Many people with acute sinusitis are able to recover completely without taking antibiotics. Simple self-care and over-the-counter medications are often all that are needed:

- *Drink plenty of fluids to keep nasal discharge thin.* The sinuses drain more easily when they are well hydrated. Water is an essential nutrient. Drink eight to ten 8-ounce glasses a day—even more when you are physically active. Healthy beverages such as natural fruit juices or herbal teas can substitute for water, but avoid sugary drinks, alcohol, and caffeinated beverages. Spread your liquid intake throughout the day.

• *Get adequate rest.* A lack of sleep may weaken your immune system and make you more susceptible to colds and sinus infections. It's also important to pace yourself and not overdo during the acute phase of an infection. Getting restorative sleep is essential.

• *Have a home steam treatment.* Inhaling steam can relieve some of the discomfort of sinusitis, colds and flu, sore throats, and laryngitis. The moisture in the steam helps loosen secretions in the nose, throat, and lungs, making them easier to clear. Try taking a hot shower or running hot water while you are in the bathroom, and inhale the steam. Alternatively, fill a bowl a third full with hot water, lean forward, pull a towel completely over your head and the bowl, and inhale the steam for several minutes.

• *Apply warm compresses.* Like steam, warm and moist towels applied over the face can help relieve congestion by allowing the sinuses to drain. As an added dividend, they're very soothing and relaxing.

• *Place a humidifier in your bedroom.* This will keep your mucous membranes from becoming dry and irritated. Humidifiers are especially important in dry winter months.

• *Sleep with your head elevated.* Sleep on a wedge with a pillow on top of it. Also try to sleep on your side with the uninfected sinus down toward the pillow. This will permit the sinuses on the upper side to drain.

• *Gently blow your nose, blocking one nostril while blowing through the other.* Avoid violent nose blowing, which can lead to physical damage and further blockage.

• *Avoid air pollutants, strong fumes, secondhand smoke, and cold or dry air.* These can cause further inflammation and irritation, as well as defects in mucociliary activity. If exposure is unavoidable, wear a protective mask over your nose and mouth.

• *Use an oral decongestant such as Sudafed or a nasal spray decongestant such as Neosynephrine or Afrin.* These over-the-counter remedies constrict blood supply to mucous membranes, resulting in less swelling, a decreased volume of blood, and reduced resistance to nasal airflow. However, they have serious side effects such as insomnia and should not be used if you have hypertension or an enlarged prostate. In addition, nasal spray decongestants cannot be used for more than three days, or they will cause a rebound effect.

■ *Irrigate the nose and sinuses.* Commercial saline sprays can help you breathe easier by clearing the sinuses of thickened secretions and crusty debris. Alternatively, make your own nasal irrigation rinse with a quart of tap or bottled water, two to three teaspoons of additive-free salt, and a teaspoon of baking soda. Store for up to a week, and shake before using.

HELPFUL EQUIPMENT AND PRODUCTS

Hordes of products purport to control sinusitis and sinus-related diseases such as allergies and asthma. Some of these devices are useful, while others are a waste of your money. The following products are generally recommended:

■ *"Green" Cleaning Products* Strongly scented cleaning products can irritate the sinuses and act as a trigger of allergic rhinitis in many people. Environmentally sound "green" cleaning products are less dependent on harsh chemicals and are usually available unscented. Safe and natural cleaning substances include baking soda, distilled white vinegar, lemon juice, and borax. Alternatively, designer retailers such as Conran's, Crate & Barrel, and Williams-Sonoma offer aromatherapy cleaning products, including Caldrea, Method, and Mrs. Meyer's. Instead of harsh chemical scents, these feature aromas like basil, lavender, citrus, and green apple. Yet be careful—just like perfumes, these scents too can cause allergic symptoms in some people.

■ *Humidifiers* Like steam treatments, humidifiers are good sources of moist air. They are particularly helpful in the cold winter months, when you have the heat on, the windows closed, and your dry and irritated sinus membranes are in desperate need of moisture. If you have a sinus infection, use a humidifier every night to relieve coughing and sore throat. To create a moist environment, turn on a humidifier near your bed and close the bedroom door. Warm humidifiers are generally preferable to cool ones, as they are more sterile. But whatever type of device you choose, it is still necessary to wash its tank weekly with vinegar water. Otherwise, the humidifier becomes a breeding ground for mold and bacteria that can then recirculate into the air.

- *Dehumidifiers* While too little moisture can impair drainage by drying out and irritating delicate mucous membranes, too much moisture in the air may lead to the development of troublesome mold spores that can provoke symptoms. To avoid this situation, keep the humidity in your home below 50 percent. If necessary, install dehumidifiers in a damp basement or bathroom. (Remember to clean their collecting pans on a regular basis.)
- *HVAC: Heating, Ventilation, and Air-Conditioning Systems* The quality of the air you breathe in your home is dependent upon the quality of these systems. To ensure clean air, maintain these systems well. As they grow older, air conditioners can benefit from a yearly tune-up. Change the filters on a regular basis, and consider investing in an air filtration system. These can be part of your HVAC system, or you can buy stand-alone air cleaners.
- *Air Filters or Purifiers* Electronic air cleaners clean household air and produce positive ions. Many of the best ones use HEPA (High Efficiency Particle Accumulation) filters. These filters can absorb and remove more than 99 percent of particles in the air—including dust mites, pollen, viruses, bacteria, mold spores, tobacco smoke, odors, particulate air pollution, and dog and cat hair and dander. ULPA (Ultra Low Penetration Air) filters are even more efficient. Air conditioners and vacuum cleaners should be equipped with good HEPA or ULPA filters. Check and change them on a regular basis.

SELF-CARE FOR COLDS

Because acute sinusitis most frequently follows a cold, it is important to prevent upper respiratory infections. Colds are more common in the chilly winter months—not because viruses thrive in this weather, but due to the fact that we spend so much time indoors, passing our germs back and forth to one another. Fortunately, there are many things you can do to avoid getting a cold. These same strategies can also keep you from passing on your own cold germs to others—especially those who are prone to sinusitis. To contain contagious airborne viruses, try the following:

- Wash your hands frequently, especially after sneezing or blowing your nose. A virus can remain on your hands for hours, so try not to touch your face or bite your nails.

- Turn away from others when you cough or sneeze.
- Use tissues instead of handkerchiefs. (Tissues with lotion or aloe are easier on tender noses.)
- Use paper cups and paper towels in bathrooms.
- Do not share eating utensils with others.
- When using the telephone (especially a public phone), avoid direct contact with the receiver.
- Keep sick children home from day care or school.

If, despite these precautions, you still come down with a cold, the following measures may be beneficial:

- Drink plenty of clear liquids, such as water, broth, juice, and tea. Warm liquids are especially soothing.
- Avoid alcohol and caffeine, which contribute to dehydration by drawing water from cells.
- Cut back on heavy, fatty foods and dairy products, which increase mucous production.
- Don't smoke. Not only does smoking inhibit your body's ability to fight disease, it also weakens the mucous barrier and aggravates your cough.
- Get plenty of rest—this will help you fight off a cold.
- Limit yourself to light exercise only.
- Avoid stress, which weakens your immune defenses.
- To breathe more easily, sleep with your head elevated.
- Use humidifiers or steam treatments to prevent dry mucous membranes.
- Take over-the-counter medication to relieve the day-to-day discomfort of colds and coughs.

SELF-CARE FOR ALLERGIES

Like colds, allergies may precipitate sinus disease—so controlling your allergies can prevent an acute episode of sinusitis from developing. It is essential to learn to identify the triggers of your symptoms. These vary from person to person, but may include mold, dust, and pollen. Next, identify situations that bring you into contact with your triggers, and devise strategies to avoid them.

In Your Home

If you or someone you live with is prone to allergies or sinusitis, it is important to keep your home as dirt-free and orderly as possible. Helpful strategies include:

- Thoroughly clean your house on a regular basis.
- Have someone else do the vacuuming, or wear a mask when you do it.
- Install an air filter or purifier to clean household air.
- Keep humidity below 50 percent to prevent the development of mold spores.
- When your house needs a fresh coat of paint, have someone else do the job. Paint fumes can trigger allergies. Whatever you do, don't sleep in a freshly painted room.
- Avoid using toxic chemicals or pesticides.
- Do not use air fresheners or potpourri.
- Avoid decorating your home with too many fussy knick-knacks, which are an invitation to dust.
- Install air-conditioning to lessen exposure to allergens.
- To prevent mold growth, limit the number of indoor plants.
- If you have pets, at least ban them from the bedroom.

Coping with Animal Allergens

Household pets such as dogs, cats, hamsters, rabbits, and birds all produce dander, an amalgam of tiny traces of their saliva, urine, and feces. Pet dander is a potent trigger of congestion, sneezing, and other symptoms, so try these measures to control animal allergens:

- Keep certain areas of the home (especially your bedroom) pet- and dander-free.
- Keep pets outside as often as possible.
- Wash your animals and have them groomed on a regular basis.
- Vacuum frequently to remove pet hair.
- Avoid placing pesticide-laden flea collars on pets. Pesticides are potent triggers of allergies. Instead, look for natural flea controls, which are available at most pet stores. (They're also safer for your pet.)
- Install HEPA-quality air filters on vacuum cleaners and air conditioners, and consider investing in an air purifier.

Control the Cockroach Population

Cockroach droppings—one of the more unpleasant components of house dust—can trigger allergic reactions and asthma attacks. In fact, asthma is rising to epidemic proportions in inner-city children, who are routinely exposed to pollutants, dust, and cockroaches. Take these steps to control cockroach infestations:

- Hire an exterminator to fumigate your home. Leave the apartment or house during this process, and stay away for several hours. When you come back, immediately open the windows and doors for ventilation.
- Following extermination, clean your home thoroughly. Carefully wipe all surfaces.
- To prevent reinfestation, seal off any cracks.
- Set out roach traps.
- Keep your home as clean as possible. Pay special attention to the kitchen. Don't leave food out and make sure dirty dishes don't accumulate in the sink. Empty garbage on a regular basis, and get rid of old newspapers.

Beware of Dust Mites

House dust is a mixture of organic and inorganic materials such as skin cells shed by people and animals, tiny bits of food, and pollen. Most people are not allergic to house dust itself, but rather to the dust mites that thrive upon it. Dust mites—tiny eight-legged insects that live on dead skin flakes, hair, nails, bacteria, fungi, and animal dander—are one of the largest causes of year-round allergies. Their waste is an especially potent component of house dust. Dust mites thrive in dark, warm, and humid conditions. In your home, these tiny creatures burrow deep into carpets, upholstered furniture, soft toys, and bedding. Following are some helpful techniques to control house dust and dust mites:

- Dust and mop regularly with damp or treated cloths (such as Pledge Grab-Its), which efficiently remove dust rather than just spreading it around.
- Use a strong, canister-style machine to vacuum.
- If an expensive vacuum cleaner is not in your budget, use high-efficiency dust bags. While they cost more than standard

bags, high-efficiency bags contain electrostatically charged fibers that trap far more dust.

- Vacuuming raises dust particles, which remain in the air for about an hour afterward. Once again: install a filter on your vacuum cleaner, ask someone else to vacuum for you, or wear a mask while you do the job.
- Vacuum not only the rug, but also the floor, upholstered furniture, curtains, and pillows.

Banish Dust Collectors from Your Home

If you are susceptible to allergies and sinusitis, it's best to keep clutter to a minimum. A house filled with fussy knickknacks is an open invitation to dust and dust mites. Use these strategies to keep your home clean and simple:

- Eliminate elaborate decorations and furnishings.
- Remove wall-to-wall carpeting. Plain wood or linoleum floors are the best way to allergy-proof your home. If you prefer to have rugs, opt for throw rugs that you can launder frequently.
- Replace heavy drapes with light, easily washable ones—or consider using shades only.
- Simply painted walls are best. Wallpaper and fabric-covered walls are dust collectors.

Allergy-Proof Your Bedroom

People spend about a third of their lives in the bedroom, and your bed is one of the dust mite's favorite haunts. Mattresses, box springs, pillows, and stuffed animals can provide nesting space for literally millions of these microscopic annoyances. Fortunately, there are many strategies to allergy-proof your bedroom:

- To keep your room dust-free, wash bedding weekly in very hot water (at least 130 degrees).
- Air out bedding on a regular basis.
- Encase mattresses, box springs, duvets, and pillows in airtight covers.
- Avoid down-filled pillows and comforters; synthetic materials such as nonallergenic Dacron pillows are less apt to disturb

allergies. Foam pillows are another poor alternative, as perspiration may make them grow moldy.

- Replace your pillows every year or two.
- Use undyed cotton sheets.
- Instead of wool or down covers, opt for blankets made of washable nylon.
- Remove dust collectors such as wall-to-wall carpeting, heavy curtains, and upholstered furniture.
- Keep items such as pictures, photos, shelves, and decorative pillows to a minimum. Bare surfaces are less hospitable to dust and dust mites.
- Keep your bedroom closet neat and orderly. Do not allow clothing or clutter to accumulate on the floor. Keep the closet door closed.
- If you want bookshelves in your bedroom, consider the kind with glass windows.
- Do not store items under your bed.
- Clean floors regularly with a damp mop.
- Vacuum thoroughly once a week. If this aggravates your allergies, wear a mask.
- On a periodic basis, use a superheated steam cleaner to remove dust, animal dander, and mold spores.
- Use window shades instead of heavy drapes or blinds.
- If your bedroom is damp, use a dehumidifier to keep humidity under 50 percent. If it is dry, a humidifier can help you breathe more easily. (Most devices come with a gauge to help you maintain humidity at an appropriate level.)
- Cover heating vents with filters.
- If you can't afford central air-conditioning throughout the house, try to at least install a single air conditioner in the bedroom.
- If pollen triggers your allergies, keep the windows closed and the air conditioner on during pollen season.
- In a child's bedroom, limit stuffed animals to a few washable ones.
- Make your bedroom off-limits to pets.

Allergy-Proof Your Bathroom, Kitchen, and Basement

Mold (also known as mildew) thrives in damp environments such as the bathroom and basement. In the kitchen, gas emitted by the stove is a powerful pollutant, while food residue attracts cockroaches. Although you may be tempted to use strongly scented cleaning products to vanquish these foes, strong odors, too, can trigger allergic symptoms. Instead, try these strategies:

- Make certain that your bathroom, kitchen, and basement are well ventilated. After you take a shower or bath, open the window a crack to allow moisture to dissipate.
- Clean any visible mold using a nonchlorine bleach.
- Scrub bathroom tiles and fixtures on a regular basis. Replace shower curtain liners as necessary.
- Don't use scented soaps.
- Whenever possible, open a window before turning on gas burners in the kitchen.
- Keep your refrigerator neat and clean. Watch expiration dates, and promptly remove any spoiled food.
- Take out the trash on a regular basis, and keep the trash container clean.
- To discourage mold growth, repair any leaks in the basement.
- Install dehumidifiers as necessary.
- Instead of using strongly scented cleaning products, choose natural alternatives such as baking soda, distilled white vinegar, lemon juice, and borax. New aromatherapy cleaning products—such as green tea and patchouli dish soap—are available at upscale retailers including Conran's, Crate & Barrel, and Williams-Sonoma.

Around Your Yard and Garden

To a person who suffers from seasonal or mold allergies, working around the yard can be like negotiating a dangerous minefield. Pollution and pesticide residues also pose problems in the great outdoors. Following are some tips on how to avoid them:

- If you're allergic to pollen, call the American Lung Association for a guide to the seasonal patterns in your area. (When you travel, it's also a good idea to get an idea of the pollen count you can expect at your destination.)
- Check your newspaper for the daily pollen count. When it's on the low side, it's safe to spend time outdoors. But when

warnings are issued that the pollen count is up, stay indoors, close the windows, and turn on the air-conditioning.

- If you live in an urban area where pollution is a problem, check the daily news about the ozone count or pollution levels. If they're high, avoid spending time outdoors. Stay indoors with the windows closed and the air-conditioning on.
- If you're allergic to mold, keep your yard on the dry side. Don't plant dense vegetation near the house. In the fall, have someone else to rake the leaves. Quickly remove piles of rotting leaves, which are open invitations to mold spores. For the same reason, do not keep a compost pile.
- If cut grass triggers your allergies, arrange for someone else to cut your lawn. If this isn't possible, at least wear a mask when you do the job.
- Do not use pesticides on your lawn or garden. Instead of these potent allergens, look for natural alternatives. For instance, certain flowers naturally repel insects.
- If cold air triggers allergy or asthma symptoms, in cold weather wear a scarf to cover your nose and mouth. If you know in advance that you will be exposed to cold air (for instance, when you're going skating or skiing), ask your doctor about prescribing preventive medication.

Eliminate Airborne Irritants

Airborne irritants—such as tobacco smoke, house dust, mold spores, animal dander, and pollen—are among the most common triggers of allergies. Try these tips to remove irritating substances such as these from your environment:

- Make your home a smoke-free zone.
- Install air-conditioning to limit your exposure to allergens.
- Use an electrostatic filter in the air conditioner to remove pollutants from household air. Replace filters frequently—otherwise, you just recirculate polluted air.
- If you don't have central air-conditioning, consider stand-alone air purifiers.
- Monitor humidity levels in your home.
- When seasonal allergies are acting up, close the windows and turn the air-conditioning on.

- Avoid using pesticides, harsh cleaning chemicals, paint fumes, perfumes, etc.

When You Travel

As with any other aspect of travel, good preparations health-wise can make your trip go more smoothly. For example, if pollen triggers your symptoms, check in advance what the pollen count will be at your destination. Keep medications close at hand, but also bring backup prescriptions just in case you misplace them. In addition, try these helpful strategies:

- If you have allergies, always keep your personal triggers in mind, and take appropriate steps to avoid them. For instance, if pollution has been associated with past cases of allergic reactions and subsequent sinusitis, don't choose to visit polluted areas.
- Choose clean and well-maintained places to stay.
- In hotels and motels, make sure you book a nonsmoking room.
- Ask to see your room before you pay for it. If there is dust, mildew, or an odor of stale cigarette smoke, switch to a different room, or move to another hotel.
- If you are allergic to feathers, bring your own pillow.
- If your allergies are especially severe, consider traveling with a portable HEPA air filter system.
- On the road, if pollutants or pollen is troublesome, keep the windows closed and the air-conditioning on. Instead of opening the vent to outside air, choose the air conditioner setting that recirculates cool air through the car.
- Don't allow anyone to smoke in the car.
- Take advantage of clean rest stops. Avoid using dirty, moldy bathrooms in service stations.
- If certain foods or food additives cause allergic reactions, be especially careful when you order meals (especially in foreign countries). Order simple, recognizable items.
- In case of emergency, wear a Medic Alert pendant or bracelet. Ask your doctor to write out any special instructions for emergency treatment.

On the Airplane

Airplanes are virtual petri dishes for microorganisms. Their cabins are tightly sealed, lack adequate air filtering, and are often inadequately cleaned. It is best to avoid air travel when you are actively suffering from cold or allergy symptoms. If you must fly at those times, take a decongestant before descent to prevent sinus blockage and to allow mucus to drain. Whenever you are planning to travel by air, try these tips:

- Keep your medication in your carry-on bag—not in the baggage compartment, where it can do you no good if symptoms occur during the flight.
- Keep all medications in their original containers. Not only will this make it easier and less confusing for you (or someone else who needs to give you medication), it will also make customs officials less suspicious.
- Drink plenty of water. Avoid alcohol and caffeinated beverages, which are dehydrating.
- If possible, upgrade to business or first class to give yourself a little more personal space. On long flights, periodically get up and stretch and walk around.
- If you habitually experience severe pain during the pressure changes of air travel, see your doctor. You may have sinus obstruction.
- Most domestic airlines now ban smoking. But whenever you book an international flight on a foreign airline or a charter, make sure no smoking is permitted.
- If you have food allergies, order a special fruit or vegetarian meal in advance. Regular airline food is packed with chemicals and preservatives.

Control Food Allergies

Common food allergens include peanuts, shellfish, eggs, cow's milk products, and wheat. Strict avoidance is the best way to control allergies that are related to food and food additives. Once you have identified the substances that cause problems for you, try the following strategies to eliminate them from your diet:

- Read labels carefully. Often, canned or prepared products contain small amounts of substances to which you may be sensitive or allergic.
- When in doubt about ingredients at a supermarket or grocery store, request further information.
- If you are sensitive to certain foods or food additives (such as sulfites, tartrazine, or MSG), don't hesitate to ask at restaurants if they have been used in the preparation of the dishes you would like to order.
- If you're sensitive to sulfites, avoid consuming wine, beer, dried fruits, and processed foods. Also be careful at salad bars, where sulfites are often added to prevent discoloration and keep greens looking greener.
- Beware of potential allergens in related food groups. For instance, if you are allergic to milk, you should also avoid eating dairy products such as yogurt and cheese.
- If your child has food allergies, alert his or her school. Some schools actually ban allergy-provoking foods such as peanut products, or at least establish peanut butter–free zones in the lunchroom.
- If agricultural chemicals trigger allergic reactions, choose free-range, hormone-free, and organic food products.
- If your food allergies are severe, wear a Medic Alert pendant or bracelet, and ask your doctor to prescribe an epinephrine kit such as EpiPen.

MAINTAIN A HEALTHY LIFESTYLE

When all is said and done, never underestimate the power of a simple, healthy lifestyle. A well-balanced diet can help maintain normal mucous flow, while drinking lots of water hydrates the sinuses. Both primary and secondary exposure to smoke contributes to sinus problems and should be strictly avoided at all times. It's also essential to get a proper balance of exercise and rest. Steps like these can enhance your immune system, boost your energy, and make you feel better overall.

- *Follow a healthy diet.* A well-balanced diet emphasizes fruits and vegetables, whole grains, legumes, nuts, and fish. Several servings a day of fruits, vegetables, and whole grains provide not only valuable dietary fiber but also antioxidant nutrients that strengthen your immune system. A good diet also means one that is low in saturated fat, cholesterol, sodium, and sugar. This means moderating your consumption of animal products such as meat, poultry, eggs, and whole milk foods. It's also important to limit your intake of caffeine-packed coffee or diet soda, and sugar-laden cookies and cakes. Sugar provides an initial burst of energy, but is soon followed by a crash. Research has also shown that a daily glass of wine can benefit your health, but consistently drinking more than this can be damaging. Nearly everyone can benefit from taking a daily vitamin and mineral supplement. If you have food allergies, it is important to identify and eliminate any troublesome foods from your diet.

▪ *Don't smoke, and limit your exposure to environmental tobacco smoke.* It would be hard to overestimate the health risks posed by smoking. Cigarette smoke contains over four thousand chemicals, dozens of which are carcinogenic. Environmental tobacco smoke—a major indoor air pollutant—is associated with airway inflammation. Smoking when you have sinusitis can worsen the infection. The good news is that most adult smokers say they want to quit. While quitting is difficult, your chances of breaking the habit are greater today than ever before, thanks to a variety of support groups and quit-smoking programs, as well as medications. Many people find nicotine inhalers or patches beneficial.

▪ *Reduce your exposure to indoor and outdoor pollutants.* Scientists agree that sinus-related disease is on the rise worldwide and is related to an increase in urban air pollution. Particles and gases in outdoor air irritate delicate sinus tissue, while indoor air pollution poses even more serious health hazards. Check your radio or television weather reports or your local newspaper for information about air quality, and avoid vigorous outdoor activity on "ozone alert" days. If you have sinus disease—especially if it is accompanied by allergies—also wear a mask while working in the yard. One of the indoor pollutants of greatest concern is environmental tobacco smoke, which increases the risk of respiratory infections in children. In your home, also be on the lookout for other irritants that you can control, such as dust, mold, household cleansers, and scented toiletries. When you use items such as hair spray or cleaning fluid, hold your breath and leave the area until the droplets dissipate. Wear a mask when vacuuming. If you work in one of the so-called sick buildings—high-rise, airtight structures built during the 1970s energy crisis, to retain heat—beware of symptoms such as headaches, fatigue, dizziness, and trouble concentrating.

- *Get an annual flu shot.* This is especially important for people over the age of sixty-five; those with chronic medical conditions, such as asthma, diabetes, or heart disease; people who are taking immunosuppressive drugs, including chemotherapy or radiation for cancer; women who will be in the second or third trimester of pregnancy during flu season; and health workers who care for high-risk patients.

- *Get adequate sleep and regular exercise.* A good balance of rest and exercise can go far toward building up your stamina and resistance to infections. Especially when you are under stress, getting a good night's sleep is essential. To boost your energy, fill in sleep gaps with a twenty- to thirty-minute catnap in the afternoon. (Longer naps can leave you feeling woozy rather than rejuvenated.)

Exercise provides both physical and emotional health. Regular aerobic activity such as brisk walking tones your heart and the blood vessels that carry blood from your heart to all the vital organs of your body. Exercise also imparts a general sense of well-being, reduces stress, and helps you get a good night's sleep. All kinds of exertion are good for you. However, if you have an active case of sinusitis, ask your doctor whether it would be better for you to at least temporarily avoid swimming.

- *Know the symptoms of sinus disease.* Nasal congestion, headaches, facial pain, and other sinusitis symptoms are not normal. If you experience problems like these, see your doctor.

Natural Sleep Strategies

Sleeping pills can be habit-forming, and doctors do not recommend using them for more than a short period of time. Instead, try these natural sleep strategies:

- Do not use your bed for activities such as working on the laptop or watching TV. Reserve it for sleep. If you're tossing and turning, go into another room and read, sip a cup of herbal tea, or otherwise relax for half an hour. Then go back to bed.
- Be sure you have a comfortable bed and supportive pillow. If you are suffering from sinus disease, sleep with your head elevated.

- Keep your bedroom dark and quiet. If necessary, use a white-noise generator or tapes of nature sounds such as the ocean or falling rain to block out street noise.
- To establish normal sleep rhythms, go to bed at night and get up in the morning at the same time every day (even on weekends).
- In the hour before retiring, avoid overly stimulating activity such as vigorous exercise, listening to loud music, or playing computer games. Don't read material from work or watch the evening newscast just before going to bed.
- Especially if you have reflux disease, avoid consuming caffeine, alcohol, or rich foods in the late evening.
- Establish a regular, comforting, wind-down routine, such as a warm relaxing bath or a quiet hour of light, recreational reading.
- If you still can't get a good night's sleep, see your doctor.

WHEN SELF-CARE IS NOT ENOUGH

Clearly, there are dozens of steps that you can take to harness your body's natural defenses to prevent or lessen the symptoms of sinusitis and related diseases. As you will see in the next chapter, some people also move beyond these simple self-care strategies to explore alternative therapies such as acupuncture or herbal remedies. Always keep in mind, however, that severe or persistent cases of sinusitis require medical evaluation and treatment.

CHAPTER 10

Complementary and Alternative Therapy

Fully one-third of the people in the United States have tried some form of complementary or alternative therapy. Perhaps because chronic sinus disease can be so frustrating to cope with, many sinus sufferers number among those who turn to complementary approaches such as acupuncture, aromatherapy, herbal therapy, homeopathy, hydrotherapy, nutritional supplements, reflexology, and relaxation techniques.

COMPLEMENTARY OR ALTERNATIVE: WHAT'S THE DIFFERENCE?

Although the two terms are most often used synonymously, some experts make a distinction between complementary and alternative therapy. Complementary therapy is said to take place *in addition* to standard medical treatment, while alternative medicine *replaces* standard treatment. If viewed in this context, complementary would naturally be a safer choice than alternative therapy.

A GROWING ACCEPTANCE

Not too long ago, complementary remedies were thought to belong solely in the realm of quacks, fanatics, and crackpots. But in recent years, there has been a growing acceptance that they can play a valuable role in the healing process. From the standpoint of consumers, complementary medicine offers an attractive alternative to managed care. Many sinus sufferers—as well as other patients—feel that they no longer get as much time and personal attention from their doctors. This may be one reason why people are turning in droves to alternative practitioners, who generally are able to spend more time with their patients and take a more holistic and compassionate approach to healing. From a doctor's perspective, nearly every medical school in this country now has courses on complementary medicine. Moreover, in 1992, the National Institutes of Health (NIH) established the National Center for Complementary and Alternative Medicine. At the American Academy of Otolaryngology–Head and Neck Surgery, a Committee on Alternative Medicine has been formed to serve as a source of information for physician members.

BUYER BEWARE

Although there are many legitimate alternative medical practices out there, at present it's still up to you as the consumer to separate the wheat from the chaff. The best approach is caveat emptor: "Let the buyer beware." If it sounds too good to be true, it probably is. But the problem confounding consumers and doctors alike is the scarcity of good scientific research to back up sometimes reasonable—and other times extravagant—claims. At present there are few valid studies of alternative approaches. Even when research exists, it tends to be from spotty studies that are too small or of poor quality. This is at least partly due to the way that alternative therapies are regulated in this country. For example, an herbal remedy—unlike a drug—cannot be patented by any one company in the United States. This gives manufacturers little incentive to spend millions of dollars on costly studies. With the growing interest in alternative approaches, and the commitment of government agencies such as the NIH, this situation may change. In the meantime, take reasonable precautions to protect yourself.

SAFETY FIRST

Although people are turning, in record numbers, to one sort of alternative relief or another, many are hiding this fact from their doctors. Don't make this mistake, which can pose serious risks to your health. It is essential for your physician to know about all medications that you take, whether they are prescription, over-the-counter, or alternative. Just like more conventional drugs, complementary remedies can have side effects and dangerous interactions with other chemical substances. To be on the safe side, always take the following precautions before using any alternative remedy:

- Make certain that you have a correct diagnosis of your medical problem.
- Tell your doctor about the natural remedy you are considering. Discuss its risks, benefits, side effects, and possible interaction with any other drugs you are taking.
- Look carefully into the pros and cons of a product before trying it. Do your homework: Are there any data to substantiate its claims?
- Do not stop taking your regular medication without talking to your doctor.
- Keep in mind that natural is not synonymous with safe, and maintain a healthy degree of skepticism.

DIFFERENT TYPES OF COMPLEMENTARY THERAPIES

Complementary and alternative therapies are many and varied. Some are beneficial, while others do indeed fit the definition of quackery. In the section that follows, we examine some popular alternative approaches to sinusitis.

ACUPUNCTURE AND ACUPRESSURE

These ancient Chinese practices are based on the theory that your body has a natural flow of energy or life force known as *qi* (pronounced "chee"). According to holistic experts, *qi* flows through the body along fourteen primary pathways known as meridians. When *qi* gets blocked along one of these paths, pain or disease—such as sinusitis—may result. Unblocking these channels using acupuncture or acupressure may provide relief.

When you visit an acupuncturist, extremely fine steel needles are lightly inserted into specific points on your skin. These needles are then rotated by hand, or an electric current is applied to them. The goal is to balance the flow of *qi*. Although many people are uncomfortable with the idea of these needles, in fact they are so thin that there is usually only minor discomfort.

Another alternative is acupressure, which works in a similar way. However, rather than using needles, the practitioner uses his or her hands to stimulate certain points on the skin. Applying pressure to these points for three to five minutes is said to unblock meridians and restore the proper flow of *qi*. This in turn would theoretically relieve the symptoms of sinusitis.

Many people swear by acupuncture and acupressure. Alas, there are very few studies that evaluate its efficacy, and those that exist are often flawed. In one small study of six patients, acupuncture was of no benefit to severe sinus sufferers, and all eventually underwent surgery.

IS ACUPUNCTURE SAFE?

Since dangerous diseases such as hepatitis are transmitted by dirty needles, it's natural to feel some degree of concern about the safety of acupuncture. But the surgical steel needles that are used in this practice are sterile, individually wrapped, and disposable. This makes infection highly unlikely.

To make sure that you are getting the best and safest care, choose a practitioner who has the proper credentials. Acupuncturists can receive certification from the American Academy of Medical Acupuncturists, the American Association of Oriental Medicine, and/or the National Commission for the Certification of Acupuncture. (Many states also offer certification.) Call one of these organizations for referral to a certified acupuncturist in your area.

AROMATHERAPY

Aromatherapy is the art of using essential oils to enhance your health and well-being. Essential oils distilled from plants, flowers, trees, fruits, and herbs have been prized since ancient times for their impact on the body and mind. There is even a certain amount of science to back this up. The olfactory nerve—the nerve involved in smell—connects with some of the most powerful parts of the brain. Recent studies have shown positive effects of aromatherapy on anxiety, skin conditions, pain, blood pressure, headaches, cigarette craving, and even computational speed. While there is no specific research on aromatherapy and sinusitis, it stands to reason that by promoting a sense of well-being, aromatherapy may decrease susceptibility to upper respiratory infections and bacterial sinusitis. Certain scents are also believed to help clear up sinus congestion.

Aromatherapy for sinusitis might include the following:

- Eucalyptus—a popular ingredient in many conventional cold and sinus remedies—has a fresh and pungent scent that can be inhaled several times a day to help relieve sinus congestion. Partially fill a large bowl with a quart of hot water, add three drops of the essential oil of eucalyptus, cover your head with a towel, and rest your head about twelve inches above the water. Inhale the steam for several minutes.
- At night, place a bowl of hot water containing one drop of eucalyptus and three drops of benzoin by your bed. Benzoin has a soothing, warm vanilla scent. The combination of these two essential oils may help clear stuffy sinuses, contribute to your relaxation, and help you get a good night's sleep.
- Mix one drop of eucalyptus with a tablespoon of a vegetable carrier oil. Apply this mixture to your chest, or use it to gently massage the sinus area. (Never directly apply undiluted essential oils to your skin, as they are very strong and may cause a rash. Good carrier oils are available from the same sources as essential oils—visit a local health food store you trust, or contact the American Aromatherapy Association, Institute of Classical Aromatherapy, National Association for Holistic Aromatherapy, or Pacific Institute of Aromatherapy for further information.)
- Other potentially beneficial essential oils include cypress, mint, Roman chamomile, and thyme.

HERBAL THERAPY

Herbal therapy is the use of healing remedies prepared from the roots, leaves, and other parts of plants. Its holistic outlook emphasizes

AROMATHERAPY CLEANING PRODUCTS

Aromatherapy is now available for your home as well as your body. A number of new upscale cleaning products—from dish soaps to window cleaners—are now available in scents such as grapefruit, lavender, lemon verbena, pine, and rosemary. (Turn back to chapter 9 to read more about these products.)

promoting health and preventing disease. The use of herbs is one of the hottest alternative approaches, with sales skyrocketing since the early 1990s. Herbal remedies once occupied a quiet niche in the health store; their manufacture is now a multibillion-dollar industry, and you can find an aisle of herbal remedies in most drugstores.

Herbal Remedies Are Poorly Regulated

In 1994, the Dietary Supplement Health and Education Act (DSHEA) categorized herbs as supplements, thus exempting them from the regulations that govern prescription and over-the-counter medications. As long as a product's ingredients were on the market prior to 1994, an herbal manufacturer is not required to provide the Food and Drug Administration with the product's safety profile. Thus, it is up to the FDA to prove that a drug is unsafe, rather than the manufacturer to prove that it is safe. As a result, questions arise only after a number of adverse reactions have been reported to the FDA.

Choose Herbs Wisely

At least partly due to such lax regulation, the quality of alternative remedies varies widely from one manufacturer to another. You may be getting what it says on the label, and then again you may not. In an FDA analysis of the popular herb ginseng, there was up to a tenfold variation in the amount of the active ingredient, although all

HERBS AND MODERN MEDICINE

Herbal therapies have been the basis of many conventional drugs. Indeed, 60 percent of the best-selling prescription drugs come from natural products. For example, in chemotherapy, the popular new designer estrogen Taxol is derived from the Pacific yew tree. Looking back, aspirin originated from the bark of willow trees, digitalis from foxglove, and opiates from poppies.

were labeled as containing the same amount. Even more alarming is the occasional presence of ingredients not listed on the labels. In some cases, supplements are adulterated with pesticides, heavy metals, carcinogens, or unapproved drugs.

For all these reasons, it is important to purchase herbs and other remedies from the most reputable source you can find. If you visit a holistic practitioner, ask him or her for specific recommendations. Alternatively, try a number of different brands, and once you find the one that works best for you, stick with it. Some people prefer to buy natural remedies from large manufacturers with a long and proven track record in the production of more traditional vitamins and minerals.

THE FDA ISSUES A WARNING

Herbs have entered the supermarket as well as the drugstore. In the beverage aisle, it is now possible to buy juice laced with herbs such as echinacea, gingko, ginseng, kava, or Saint John's-wort. Indeed, herb-infused drinks are one of the fastest growing segments of the beverage business. But early in 2001, the FDA sent warning letters to several manufacturers that put herbs in their food and drinks. Under the law, food manufacturers are permitted to use only ingredients that are FDA-approved or are generally recognized as safe by scientists. Although the FDA took no official action, the warning should keep manufacturers on their toes regarding safety issues.

Herbs and Sinusitis

Alternative practitioners recommend herbs such as bromelain, echinacea, elder, goldenseal, and shea butter for the treatment of sinusitis and related illnesses:

- Several studies dating back to the 1960s indicate that bromelain—an enzyme derived from pineapple—reduces inflammation and thus improves the symptoms of sinusitis. Do not use bromelain if you are pregnant. Because it affects blood clotting, this herb should be avoided before any type of surgery (including dental).
- One of the most popular herbal remedies, echinacea is reputed to have a positive effect on the common cold. The German Commission E—a well-respected herbal authority worldwide—

rates *Echinacea purpurea* and *E. pallida* above *E. angustifolia.* Alternative practitioners advise taking echinacea at the first sign of a cold and continuing to use it for the cold's duration. It is possible that this will ease the intensity of cold symptoms and reduce their duration by several days. Experts warn people with AIDS or other autoimmune disease to avoid echinacea. Possible side effects of this herb include fever, nausea, and vomiting.

- Elder is an old country remedy for colds and flu. This herb has few side effects.
- Ginseng is said to reduce fatigue and increase stamina. It is used to lessen physical and emotional stress. However, this herb has many possible side effects and must be used with care. Its adverse reactions range from anxiety and insomnia to hypoglycemia and bleeding. Asian ginseng should not be used if you have a medical condition such as high blood pressure, and is generally not an appropriate remedy for children or premenopausal women.
- Herbalists consider goldenseal to be a natural antibiotic and immune booster. However, this herb may raise blood pressure and should not be used if you have hypertension, heart disease, or diabetes. Other possible side effects include diarrhea, hallucinations, and overexcited states. Goldenseal may also affect blood clotting. Do not use this herb if you are pregnant.
- In a small study, shea butter topically applied to the upper lip reduced nasal congestion. Shea butter, which is derived from the seed of the African shea butter tree, is generally considered safe.

Potentially Harmful Herbs

Unfortunately, some herbs have been associated with serious health problems. For example, a California woman died after taking royal bee jelly, a common herbal remedy for hay fever—it turned out she was hypersensitive to bee venom as well as pollen. Ephedra—also known as ma huang—has frequently been used as a natural nasal decongestant. However, the FDA has received more than a thousand complaints about this herb, with reports of adverse reactions such as hypertension, palpitations, seizures, and stroke. To date, seventy deaths have been associated with ephedra. Other potentially harmful herbs are listed on the next page.

Borage
Calamus
Chaparral
Coltsfoot
Comfrey
Germander
Kava
Licorice
Life root
Poke root
Sassafras

Always Consult with Your Doctor First

Just like conventional drugs, herbs have potent effects on the human body. Their active compounds may cause side effects and adverse reactions. Certain herbs are harmful if you have a preexisting condition such as high blood pressure or diabetes and, with few exceptions, herbs should be avoided during pregnancy. Plant remedies may also interact with other medications you are taking, either by reducing or adding to their effects. For your own safety, before taking any herbal remedy, always consult with your doctor.

HOMEOPATHY

Homeopathy is a system of medicine based on the principle of "like cures like." The theory is that the same substance that in large doses produces the symptoms of an illness, in very small doses cures it. Homeopathy was founded by the German physician Samuel Hahnemann in the late eighteenth century. Its development was said to be in reaction to some of the more barbaric medical practices of his day, such as bloodletting with leeches. The FDA recognizes homeopathic remedies as official drugs and regulates their manufacture, labeling, and dispensing.

Several studies have shown that homeopathic remedies may be helpful in improving allergic rhinitis symptoms and reducing the duration of flu symptoms. Oscillococcinum—a proprietary homeopathic remedy that is the largest-selling cold and flu remedy in France—in particular shows promise in limiting flu symptoms. Other homeopathic remedies for acute sinusitis include Arsenicum album, Kalium bichromium, Nux vomica, Mercurius iodatas, and Silicea.

HYDROTHERAPY

In this case, alternative practitioners are in full agreement with medical doctors: hydrotherapy such as steam inhalation, nasal irrigation, and warm compresses can all be helpful in the treatment of sinusitis. These techniques loosen nasal secretions, cleanse nasal passages, improve drainage, and allow you to breathe more easily. An herbal recipe for a nasal irrigation solution is one teaspoon of goldenseal per cup of hot water. (Read more about nasal irrigation on page 99.) To make an aromatherapeutic steam bath, fill a bowl a third full with hot water, add a drop of eucalyptus oil, drape a towel over your head, and inhale.

NUTRITIONAL SUPPLEMENTS

Many scientists believe that a proper balance of vitamins and minerals can be helpful in the treatment of any disease. Of course, like herbs and homeopathic remedies, supplements should be taken under your doctor's supervision. Two of the most frequently recommended supplements for colds—the most common precursor of acute sinusitis—are zinc products and vitamin C:

- *Zinc* Zinc is available in traditional lozenges or in a nasal gel. The new zinc-based nasal gel called Zicam shows great promise in shortening the duration of colds. However, the data on the lozenges is decidedly mixed, with pro and con studies evenly split. If you decide to give zinc a try, carefully follow the instructions on the label, and do not take more lozenges than recommended. Too much zinc can lead to nausea and vomiting, and may lower levels of HDL (the "good cholesterol"). Pregnant women should not take zinc, and studies have not yet proven the gel to be safe in children.
- *Vitamin C* There is no scientific evidence that taking vitamin C will prevent you from coming down with a cold. It is possible that large doses may reduce the duration of cold symptoms; however, large doses cause gastrointestinal problems such as diarrhea.
- *Other supplements* The human body has natural defenses against infection and tissue damage, and supplementing these defenses with a daily multivitamin can help enhance them. In addition to vitamin C, other potentially beneficial nutrients include vitamin E and beta-carotene (a precursor of vitamin A). By neu-

tralizing highly toxic molecules called free radicals, antioxidant vitamins can help prevent chronic inflammation of the sinuses.

REFLEXOLOGY

Reflexology is based on the principle that reflex areas in the hands and feet correspond to every part of the body. As a result, applying precise pressure to these areas will promote wellness. There is no clear scientific explanation why reflexology works—nevertheless, at least one recent study of chronic sinusitis suggests that it does. At the University of Wisconsin School of Medicine, a team led by Dr. Diane G. Heatley sought to determine the effect of nasal irrigation on chronic sinusitis. They recruited 150 chronic sinusitis sufferers using a newspaper advertisement. One-third used nasal irrigation with a bulb syringe; one-third used nasal irrigation with a nasal irrigation pot; and one-third used reflexology massage. The reflexology group performed daily massage on the corresponding reflex areas for the sinuses: the tips of the four fingers on both hands (excluding the thumbs) and the tips of all toes of both feet. Participants were told to apply pressure with the thumb and index finger for twenty to thirty seconds, using enough force to incur some discomfort. The results of the study were somewhat surprising. Even though the reflexology group was originally meant solely as a control, the three groups reported equally significant improvement. Symptoms improved in over 70 percent of the subjects, and medication usage was reduced in a third.

RELAXATION TECHNIQUES

Stress makes you more vulnerable to illness—moreover, the pain, anxiety, and frustration of living with a chronic disease can wreak havoc on your mind as well as your body. Quality-of-life problems posed by chronic sinusitis run the gamut from the seemingly mundane to the severe. For example, some people experience a decrease in their sense of taste and no longer enjoy eating as much as they once did. Others can't breathe well when lying down and consequently rarely get a good night's sleep. People with severe chronic sinusitis are apt to lose multiple workdays and be compelled to make repeated visits to the doctor. Some become depressed. (Read more about quality-of-life issues on pages 15–17.) Alternative approaches such as biofeedback, breathing exercises, meditation, and yoga can help you control the pain, stress, and anxiety associated with sinusitis and related problems.

Biofeedback

This technique is used for relaxation and chronic-pain management. In biofeedback, small electrodes are placed on the forehead. Through them, electronic sensors measure your body's automatic functions, such as breathing patterns, pulse rate, and muscles that contract due to tension. As you practice a relaxation method such as visualization (forming a mental image to help relax, concentrate, or cope with fear), feedback from the sensors shows whether or not you are successfully controlling your body's automatic functions. The theory is that by watching this measurement and reducing the level of electrical responses on the gauge reading, you can learn to consciously relax your muscles on your own.

Breathing Exercises

Studies have shown that there are differences in the breathing of people who are relaxed and those who are anxious. When you are worrying about sinus pain and the complications it is causing in your life, you may notice that your breathing becomes more rapid and shallow. Deep breathing, on the other hand, has a calming effect on the nervous system.

To try breathing exercises, choose a quiet time in a peaceful place. Take a deep breath in, hold for a count of three, and then slowly exhale. Sit quietly, rest one hand on your stomach, and observe your breath pass in and out of your body. If your attention starts to drift, gently draw it back and continue to watch your breath passing in and out.

Meditation

It can't cure sinusitis, but meditation *can* help you seize control of related problems such as anxiety and tension. Keep in mind, too, that controlling stress is vital to pain management. The goal of meditation is to achieve a state of deep mental and spiritual relaxation while remaining awake. This technique allows you to bring together your mind, body, and spirit in order to help you find inner peace, harmony, and tranquillity. It's best to begin meditating for short periods, say, three to five minutes at a time. If you find them satisfying, you can gradually extend the length of your meditation sessions.

Types of meditation include transcendental meditation (TM) and progressive relaxation. In transcendental meditation, you focus on a single sound or word (your mantra) while you sit quietly and breathe deeply. Concentration on a single word—such as *Om*—will help you to focus and relax. Some people also find it beneficial to focus on a single sensory memory, such as sunrise on the beach or a walk through the woods.

There are many different types of progressive relaxation. If you'd like to try this technique, simply lie down on a yoga mat (or a towel) placed on the floor of a quiet, dimly lit room. Close your eyes and try to empty your mind. Then, as you breathe in, begin to visualize the muscles of your body, beginning with your face. First tighten the muscles for a moment, and then consciously relax them. Work your way all the way down your body in this manner, from the top of your head to the tips of your toes.

Yoga
The relaxing and fluid postures of yoga are also helpful in reducing stress and tension. Yoga is closely linked with all the preceding methods of relaxation. Some of the earliest tests of biofeedback were conducted on yogis (experts in the practice of yoga), who exerted effective control over automatic body functions such as heart rate. Meditative postures, or *asanas*, bring the mind into a state of stillness and focus. In *pranayama* yoga, breathing exercises help regulate one's life force, or *prana*.

THE FUTURE OF ALTERNATIVE CARE

As increasing numbers of people are diagnosed with chronic sinusitis, the interest in alternative approaches is only likely to grow. Current research has yet to keep pace with the most up-to-date developments, and chances are that there will always be some new and unproven technique on the horizon. The best you can do is to balance good common sense with current safety guidelines while keeping an open mind to new techniques, such as those we discuss in the next chapter.

CHAPTER 11

Looking Toward the Future

Recent years have witnessed great strides in the understanding, diagnosis, and treatment of sinusitis and related diseases. As their incidence continues to climb, researchers are closely examining causal factors such as the upsurge in air pollution and decreasing immunity due to antibiotic resistance. From a theoretical standpoint, scientists are zeroing in on the immune and inflammatory elements of sinusitis, no longer viewing this as primarily an infectious problem. On the technical side, nasal endoscopy has revolutionized diagnosis and surgical treatment.

But as dramatic as these recent changes have been, we may see even more extraordinary advances in the years to come. All sorts of new drugs are on the horizon, ranging from allergy drops to cold medications to antifungals. On the vaccine front, the FDA is currently reviewing an antiflu nasal spray, and one day there may be vaccines for ear infections and allergies. To counter growing antibiotic resistance, scientists are developing novel strategies such as phage therapy (the use of tiny viruses to target and kill bacteria). And genetics will play an increasing role in sinusitis as well as in a host of other diseases. With the mapping of the human genome—the complicated double strand of DNA that contains the instructions for manufacturing every cell in the body—the very process by which new drugs are developed is likely to become transformed. DNA studies will allow more accurate diagnosis, as well as the design and administration of treatment aimed at correcting basic underlying genetic defects.

ALLERGY DROPS INSTEAD OF SHOTS?

Allergy drops—already widely available in Europe—are a promising experimental treatment currently being tried by several hundred doctors around the country. An attractive alternative to shots, allergy drops are self-administered under the tongue three times a day. Much the same as traditional allergy shots, the drops are custom-made to control your individual allergies, whether they are to dust mites, mold, tobacco, animal dander, or ragweed. Over time, weakened doses of the designated allergens are introduced into your body; these doses are gradually strengthened to encourage the buildup of a proper immune response. As with injections, it takes time for immunity to build—three to five years on average. But unlike shots, drops cause no discomfort and—as they are self-administered—do not require as many trips to the doctor's office.

A NEW WEAPON AGAINST THE COMMON COLD?

The FDA is also considering the approval of a drug called Picovir (pleconaril). Although it's not a cure, the scientists who developed this medication say that it can reduce a cold's length and severity. Picovir works by attacking the rhinovirus, which is the virus responsible for causing most colds. To be effective, medication must be taken at the first warning sign of a cold. In clinical trials, Picovir shortened the duration of colds by about a day, although uncomfortable symptoms such as sneezing and congestion began to improve even sooner. Some research also suggests that Picovir makes colds less contagious.

ADVANCES IN ANTIFUNGAL DRUGS

In recent years, fungi have been increasingly associated with stubborn, resistant cases of chronic sinusitis. Fortunately, scientists are developing a number of drugs that target these organisms. FDA approval is pending for a class of antifungals derived from Spanish soil, while researchers are looking for antifungal compounds in black sponge from the Indian Ocean. Less exotically, molecular biologists are designing drugs that specifically target and attack fungi. These new drugs kill organisms by halting protein synthesis or preventing enzymes from binding to DNA.

PROBIOTICS: BENEFITING FROM THE "GOOD BACTERIA"

Another new trend has been the growing interest in foods and other products that contain probiotics—that is, living cultures of "good bacteria." Already popular in Europe, these remedies are now beginning to take hold in the United States as well. An example of "good bacteria" is lactobacillus, bacteria that naturally reside in our intestines and also appear in foods, such as yogurt, with live cultures. Researchers in Japan have found that nasal sprays containing deactivated lactobacillus improve the ability of mice to survive the flu.

VACCINE RESEARCH SURGES FORWARD

Approximately one hundred vaccines are in various stages of development in the United States today. Scientists estimate that it takes fifteen to seventeen years to create a successful vaccine—and even longer for combination drugs designed to fight more than one disease at a time. Some of the cutting-edge vaccine research sounds almost too bizarre to be believed. For example, scientists have engineered mice that produce vaccine in their milk. In the future, they hope to extend this practice into larger milk-producing animals such as goats.

Vaccine research is also taking on a variety of new conditions, including ones that aim at lowering IgE—the major antibody responsible for allergic reaction such as an itchy, runny, or stuffy nose, watery or red eyes, and sneezing. Many vaccines in development are aimed at adults rather than children. Some are traditional preventive types, while others are so-called therapeutic vaccines designed to treat rather than prevent disease. They work by strengthening the body's immune defenses. Of course, most of these vaccines are still highly experimental, and there is no certainty that they will pass muster with the Food and Drug Administration.

New Methods of Administering Vaccines

Some vaccine research focuses on developing more user-friendly methods of delivery, such as skin patches and nasal sprays. There are high hopes for a nasal-spray flu vaccine called FluMist, which is currently under review by the FDA. This vaccine may eventually make it practical to immunize children as well as adults against the flu.

On the Horizon: A Vaccine to Prevent Ear Infections in Children

A vaccine called Prevnar was introduced in February 2000 to prevent pneumococcal disease, which causes meningitis, blood poisoning, and pneumonia in young children. Although many times more expensive than most other childhood vaccines, it has not met with any significant resistance from managed-care companies. The manufacturer—American Home Products—is currently seeking FDA approval to use Prevnar to also fight ear infections in children.

AN ALARMING TREND: GROWING ANTIBIOTIC RESISTANCE

As we've mentioned earlier, scientists warn that infections of all kinds are becoming increasingly resistant to the antibiotics we prescribe to treat them. This alarming trend is directly attributable to the overuse of antibiotics. Patients request and doctors write millions of antibiotic prescriptions each year for viral upper respiratory infections—on which antibiotics have zero impact. When antibiotics are administered too often, a few strong bacteria survive and reproduce, giving rise to new generations of resistant organisms. As more and more species of bacteria grow resistant, our current arsenal of antibiotics becomes less effective in controlling them. Organizations such as the Centers for Disease Control and Prevention, the American Medical Association, and the American Academy of Pediatrics are now publicizing this trend in a strenuous effort to halt once and for all the inappropriate use of antibiotics.

Antibiotics and the Food We Eat

Since resistant bacteria can make their way into people through the food chain, scientists are also concerned about antibiotic use in livestock. More than 40 percent of the antibiotics made in this country are given to animals to prevent infection or promote growth. Over time, exposure to low doses of antibiotics can increase the number of resistant bacteria in treated animals. These microbes may then be passed on to people who handle meat or who consume under-cooked meat.

Early in 2002, there were promising signs that the poultry indus-try, at least, was beginning to bow to the concerns of public health and consumer groups. Three major companies—Perdue, Tyson, and Foster Farms—announced that they had voluntarily cut back on the antibiotics fed to healthy chickens. One company—Foster Farms— went even farther. It also agreed to turn away from using a newer class of antibiotics, called fluoroquinolones, in sick chickens. The flu-oroquinolone drug used in poultry—Baytril—is very similar to Cipro, which is used to treat human bacterial infections including food-borne illnesses (like campylobacteriosis and salmonella) and anthrax. Scientists fear that the use of this antibiotic in chickens will cause dis-ease germs to become resistant not only to Baytril but also to Cipro and other drugs in its chemical class. In response to these concerns, the FDA has (so far unsuccessfully) been trying to ban Baytril since October 2000.

As responsible scientists continue to sound the alarm about the dangers of growing antibiotic resistance, corporate consumers too have taken note. McDonald's, Wendy's, and Popeye's are all now refusing to buy chicken that has been treated with antibiotics. Never-theless, standing in the meat aisle of the supermarket, most con-sumers find it impossible to tell which package of chicken has or has not been affected. Antibiotics continue to be administered to sick birds, and when one chicken is ill, the whole flock (which may num-ber more than thirty thousand) is treated. Public-health advocates are urging the government to intervene with some meaningful legislation, such as banning Baytril and requiring farmers to report antibiotic use in animals. In the meantime, the only certain way to buy meat that has not been adulterated with antibiotics is to purchase products labeled antibiotic-free or organic.

Antibiotics and Fruit Trees

Another problem is the treatment of fruit trees with antibiotics in aerosol spray form. The purpose is to prevent or control bacterial infections—which can affect plants as well as animals. However, antibiotic residues can encourage the growth of resistant bacteria that colonize the fruit. Moreover, the spray may accidentally hit other trees and food plants and kill harmless "good bacteria"—and thus inadvertently promote the growth of tougher, drug-resistant bacteria.

Until legislation to control this practice is enacted, you may want to consider organic produce as the safest alternative.

A Proliferation of Antibacterial Products

One of the best ways to safeguard your health—and the health of others around you—is to wash your hands on a regular basis with ordinary soap. But in the United States, we have taken this simple rule to an illogical extreme. Our strong regard for hygiene has resulted in an explosion of antibacterial soaps, lotions, and cleaning products. From just a few dozen products in the 1990s, the number has mushroomed into the hundreds today. Scientists warn that using these soaps and cleansers can be counterproductive, for bacteria may become resistant to the germ-killing chemicals in them. As with antibiotics in plants and animals, the theory is that the stronger, more drug-resistant bacteria are left free to thrive when less virulent, competing organisms are killed off.

Phage Therapy: An Ancient Cure for a Modern Problem

In this age of increasing antibiotic resistance, scientists are constantly searching for new ways to treat bacterial infections. One promising alternative is phage therapy: the use of bacteriophages, or tiny viruses that attack bacteria. These viruses have been around for billions of years but were largely ignored in the modern antibiotic era. Now researchers are giving them a second look. What scientists find so attractive about phage therapy is that, unlike antibiotics, bacteriophages do not encourage bacteria to develop resistant strains. Instead, these tiny viruses produce enzymes that kill targeted bacteria by punching holes in their cell walls. Moreover, as the equivalent of "smart bombs" in the military arena, they do this without disturbing the normal bacteria needed for health. Although not yet approved by the FDA, phage therapy has great potential for treating bacterial infections such as sinusitis. Bacteriophages could also be used as a model to make new antibacterial drugs.

MAPPING THE HUMAN GENOME

In one of the most exciting developments in our time, scientists have begun to unravel the mysteries of the human genome, plunging us headlong into the brave new world of modern, genomic medicine. The human body contains over thirty thousand different genes. Lining the forty-six chromosomes in human cells, these genes contain

DESIGNING NEW ANTIBIOTICS

As bacteria grow more drug-resistant, scientists are hard at work creating newer and more effective antibiotics. One novel approach involves the development of antibiotics based on "nanotubes," disk-shaped amino acid molecules that stack themselves into tubes when they encounter bacteria. As tiny tubes spring up inside the membrane of the bacterial cell, they punch holes in it, and the cell dies as its contents spill out. So far these new antibiotics have worked only in animals, and much more testing is required before we know if they will work in humans.

instructions for making our organs, tissue, hormones, and enzymes. Unlocking their secrets—a process that is already well under way—is likely to lead to a revolution in medicine. Amazing as it was to identify all the genes in the human body, that was only the first step. Once researchers identify the genes that cause diseases, they must locate practical applications in diagnosis and treatment. Moreover, genetic research has already led to some thorny questions, such as: Do I really want to know if I am carrying the gene for a devastating disease that currently has no cure? And how will that knowledge affect my health coverage? Whatever the answers turn out to be, treatments in the future are most likely to consist of more targeted, gene-based therapies. In gene therapy, healthy genes are transplanted into the body to prevent, manage, or cure disease. Another avenue of research involves repairing defective genes in the body. Now that scientists possess the blueprints for our genes, they can also design drugs that are more specific in their targets.

The Future of Drugs

Throughout history, drugs have been developed through the process of trial and error. But all that is about to change. The mapping of the human genome will permit the faster and more economical development of new medications. By identifying the specific molecules that make a person susceptible to a particular disease, scientists will soon be able to design drugs that target only sick cells and leave healthy ones alone. Another benefit is that genetically engineered drugs can be monitored for safety and effectiveness, so tests on human (or even animal) subjects may not be necessary. Scientists believe that every doctor's office will eventually contain equipment to produce a patient's genetic profile. Just plug that information into the computer, and it will spit out the best medication. This eliminates guesswork, as the genome will allow doctors to see clearly why a drug benefits one person and not another.

Genes and Proteins
Genes are closely related to proteins. In fact, spliced together in different combinations, genes can make more than one protein. This technique has led to the emerging field of proteinomics, in which scientists are trying to match their achievement in genomics by next identifying all the proteins in the human body and how they relate to one another. As of now, available drugs target only five hundred or so of the different proteins in the body—yet our bodies contain hundreds of thousands of proteins. Proteinomics promises to be even more complicated than genomics, because proteins are more complex than genes.

Gene Therapy, Cystic Fibrosis, and Chronic Sinusitis
Scientists have already identified the mutated gene responsible for cystic fibrosis: a gene located within region q31 on chromosome 7. At present, treatment for cystic fibrosis is aimed at controlling symptoms while scientists continue to search for a cure. Research focuses on the development of strategies to treat the defective gene.

Since so many individuals with cystic fibrosis suffer from chronic sinus infections, it came as no surprise to scientists when a genetic connection was uncovered. Chronic sinusitis sufferers have a higher incidence of a copy of the defective gene responsible for cystic fibrosis, according to research at Johns Hopkins Medical Institutions, as reported by the *Journal of the American Medical Association* in October 2000. Subsequent studies have confirmed this discovery. These people do not have cystic fibrosis, which occurs only when both parents transmit the defective gene to their offspring. However, in time they may benefit from the same therapy that is being developed for individuals with cystic fibrosis.

Research may eventually identify specific genetic defects associated with chronic sinusitis and enable us to direct gene therapy at them. Although the procedure is still in the experimental stages, inserting normally functioning genes into cells in the body may one day cure all kinds of diseases. But even before cures are discovered, understanding more about how genes work will lead to more effective prevention and treatment of diseases such as sinusitis.

GLOSSARY

Abscess—A pus-filled cavity surrounded by inflamed tissue

Acute—Describing a disorder that comes on suddenly and is usually relatively severe

Acute sinusitis—A sinus infection that lasts up to four weeks, during which there is a complete resolution of symptoms

Adenoids—Masses of lymphoid tissue that lie at the back of the nose and upper part of the throat

AIDS—Acquired immunodeficiency syndrome

Airways—The tubular passages through which air moves in and out of the lungs

Allergen—A foreign protein or molecule that, when linked to a protein, triggers allergic reactions in some people. Common allergens are house dust, pollen, animal dander, and molds.

Allergic rhinitis—Inflammation of the nasal passages as the result of an allergic reaction

Allergy—Symptoms caused by a person's antibody response to a substance that does not cause symptoms in most people

AMA—The American Medical Association

Analgesic—A medication that relieves pain

Anaphylaxis—A life-threatening allergic reaction that involves difficulty breathing and dangerously low blood pressure

Anosmia—A loss of the sense of smell

Antibiotic—A drug used to fight bacterial infections

Antibody—A molecule made by the immune system to neutralize a specific antigen in the body

Antigen—A molecule that induces the formation of antibodies

Antihistamine—A drug used to control allergies by blocking the interaction of histamine with allergic receptors

Asthma—A respiratory disorder characterized by spasms and chronic inflammation of the airways, often accompanied by wheezing and shortness of breath

Atopy—A predisposition to develop allergy because of IgE antibody hyperresponsiveness

Bacteria—Single-celled microorganisms that multiply by simple division

Barotrauma—Injuries caused by rapidly changing air pressure

Bronchitis—An inflammation of the central breathing tubes in the lungs characterized by symptoms such as coughing, increased mucous production, low-grade fever, and shortness of breath

Bronchodilator—A substance that widens the airways and thus improves breathing

Bronchospasm—An irregular contraction of smooth muscles in the lung's airways, causing the airways to narrow

Cavernous sinus thrombosis—A severe orbital complication of sinusitis in which there is inflammation of the venous channels on each side of the sphenoid sinus

CDC—The Centers for Disease Control and Prevention

Cellulitis—A bacterial infection of the skin and tissues that, left untreated, can progress to tissue damage and blood poisoning

Chemosis—Edema of the conjunctiva (the transparent mucous membrane covering the white of the eyes and lining the inside of the eyelids)

Chemotherapy—Treatment of cancer with powerful drugs

Chronic—Describing a disorder that persists for a long time

Chronic sinusitis—Sinus infection that persists for twelve weeks or longer

Cilia—Microscopic hairs that line the mucosa and propel mucus through the nasal passages and sinuses

Cold—An upper respiratory infection (URI) caused by a virus

Cold sore—A small blister around the mouth caused by the herpes simplex virus

Concha bullosa—A middle turbinate in the nose enlarged by air cells that may act as a contributing factor to sinus disease

Congestion—An excessive accumulation of fluid in body tissues

Corticosteroids—A class of drugs that are used in the treatment of inflammatory disorders

CT scan—Computerized tomography scanning

Cyst—An abnormal lump or swelling filled with fluid or semisolid material

Cystic fibrosis—A genetic disorder characterized by persistent lung infections and an inability to absorb fats and other nutrients from food

Decongestant—A drug used to relieve nasal congestion

Dura mater—The outermost layer of the three protective membranes covering and protecting the brain

Eczema—A type of inflammatory reaction of the skin

Edema—An abnormal accumulation of fluid in body tissues

Empyema—A sealed-off body cavity that contains infected matter or pus

Enzyme—A protein that acts as a catalyst to cause chemical changes in other substances but remains unchanged itself by the process

Eosinophil—A type of white blood cell that plays a role in allergic reactions

Epidural—Outside the dura mater

Epidural abscess—A collection of pus between the dura (a protective membrane surrounding the brain) and the inner surface of the skull

Ethmoid sinuses—Air-filled cavities located just behind the bridge of the nose and between the eyes

Eustachian tube—The tube that connects the middle-ear cavity to the back of the nose

Foramina—Natural openings or passages in bones or membranous structures

Frontal sinuses—Air-filled cavities located over the eyes in the brow area

Functional endoscopic sinus surgery (FESS)—Delicate sinus surgery performed with the aid of a magnified fiberoptic telescope

Fungi—Organisms that include the diverse forms of yeasts and molds

Gastroesophageal reflux—A backflow of acid from the stomach into the esophagus

Halitosis—Bad breath

Histamine—A chemical released by body cells during an allergic reaction, producing inflammation

HIV—The human immunodeficiency virus, which is the cause of acquired immunodeficiency syndrome (AIDS)

Homeostasis—The constant internal environment that is required for health, and is maintained by active processes in the body in spite of external changes

Hyposmia—A reduced sense of smell

Immunoglobulin—An antibody found in tissue fluids and serum

Immunosuppression—A reduction in the activity of the immune system

Immunotherapy—Allergy shots

Inflammation—Redness, swelling, heat, and pain resulting from the body's response to injury or infection

Inhaler—A device used to administer a drug in powder or vapor form to treat respiratory disorders

Ischemia—Decreased blood supply to an organ or tissue

Lamina papyracea—Paper-thin walls that separate the ethmoid sinuses from the orbits of the eye

Leukocyte—A white blood cell

Maxillary sinuses—Air-filled cavities that are located inside the cheekbones

Meningitis—Inflammation of the meninges (membranes that cover and protect the brain and spinal cord) that is usually bacterial, but is sometimes caused by a virus

Metabolism—The sum of the chemical processes that take place in the body

Microorganism—A tiny plant or animal life-form

MRI—Magnetic resonance imaging

Mucocele—A swollen sac or cavity filled with mucus

Mucociliary clearance—The normal production and flow of mucus in the nasal passages and sinuses that allows the nasal passages and sinuses to clear themselves of bacteria and trapped particles

Mucosa—A mucous membrane

Mucous membrane—A thin, soft, pink layer that lines many cavities and tubes in the body, including the sinuses

Mucus—A thick, slimy fluid secreted by a mucous membrane to lubricate and protect the body

Nasal cycle—The regular shrinking and swelling of the inferior turbinates, nasal septum, and ethmoid air-cell mucosa, which occurs several times a day

Nasal polyps—Mucosal sacs containing edema, fibrous tissue, vessels, inflammatory cells, and glands. They are grapelike in appearance.

Nasal septum—The central, dividing partition inside the nose

Nasopharynx—The passage connecting the cavity behind the nose to the top of the throat

Nebulizer—A device used to administer a drug in aerosol form through a face mask

Neuropathy—Disease, inflammation, or damage to one of the peripheral nerves that carry messages between the brain and spinal cord and the rest of the body

NSAIDs—Nonsteroidal anti-inflammatory drugs

Obstructed—Blocked

Ophthalmologist—A specialist in eye disorders

Ophthalmoplegia—A limited ability to move the eyes

Optic nerves—A pair of nerves that transmit information to the brain about visual images received from the retinas of the eyes

Orbit—One of the two sockets in the skull that contain the eyeballs and associated blood vessels, muscles, and nerves

Orbital abscess—A collection of pus in the orbital (eye socket) tissue

Orbital cellulitis—Infection that extends beyond the eyelid into the soft tissue of the orbit (eye socket)

Orbital subperiosteal abscess—A collection of pus between the orbit (eye socket) and the tough, fibrous membrane covering the orbital contents

Osteitis—Inflammation of bone, usually from infection

Osteomeatal unit (OMU)—An area that encompasses several middle-meatal structures into which the maxillary, frontal, and anterior ethmoid sinuses all drain. It is considered the seat of sinus disease.

Osteomyelitis—A serious infection of bones and bone marrow

Ostia—Tiny holes or openings in the sinuses through which mucus and air continuously pass

Ostial obstruction—Partial or complete blockage of the tiny holes or openings in the sinuses through which mucus and air continuously pass

Otitis media—A middle-ear infection

Otolaryngologist—A physician who has received advanced training in ear, nose, and throat disorders, including sinusitis

Palate—The roof of the mouth

Paranasal sinuses—A medical term for the sinuses, the air-filled cavities in the skull bones situated around the nose and eyes

Patent—Unobstructed

Pathogen—An organism that causes disease

Periorbita—The tough, fibrous membrane that covers the orbital contents

Periorbital cellulitis—The most common orbital complication, in which there is an abnormal infectious swelling in the eyelid

Pharyngitis—Inflammation of the pharynx; a sore throat

Pharynx—The throat; the passage that connects the back of the mouth and nose to the esophagus and trachea

Photophobia—An abnormal sensitivity to light

Postnasal drip—The flow of mucus down the back of the throat

Proptosis—Protrusion or bulging of the eyeball

Ptosis—Drooping of the upper eyelid

Purulence—Pus

Pus—A pale yellow or green creamy liquid composed of dead white blood cells and fluid that occurs at the site of a bacterial infection

RAST—Radioallergosorbent Test; a test that detects the presence in the blood of antibodies to various allergens

Recurrent acute sinusitis—Four or more episodes of acute sinusitis within one year

Respiratory system—The organs responsible for transporting oxygen from the air to the bloodstream and for expelling the waste product carbon dioxide

Retrograde thrombophlebitis—Venous inflammation with thrombus formation that propagates itself in the direction opposite to normal venous flow—that is, toward the heart

Rhinitis—Inflammation of the lining of the nose

Sick building syndrome—A collection of symptoms (such as fatigue, headache, and dry, itchy eyes) experienced by people who live or work in buildings with poor ventilation

Sinuses—Air-filled cavities in the skull bones situated around the nose and eyes

Sphenoid sinuses—Air-filled cavities located behind the ethmoid sinuses in the upper region of the nose and behind the eyes

Subacute sinusitis—Sinus infection that lasts longer than four weeks but less than twelve weeks

Subdural empyema—A collection of pus in the subdural space between the dura and the arachnoid (two of the three membranes that cover and protect the skull)

Supergerms—Also known as superbugs, bacteria that are difficult and sometimes impossible to treat with currently available antibiotics

Thrombosis—The formation of a thrombus, or blood clot, inside a blood vessel

Thrombus—A blood clot (plural: thrombi)

Tumor—An abnormal mass of tissue that develops when cells reproduce at an increased rate

Turbinate—One of three structures on the outer walls of the nasal passages on either side of the nose

Virus—A simple, tiny infectious agent that can multiply only by invading the cells of other organisms

Viscous—Thick, syrupy, and sticky

FURTHER RESOURCES

American Academy of
Otolaryngology
1 Prince Street
Alexandria, VA 22314
(703) 519-1585
www.entnet.org

American Academy of Pediatrics
141 Northwest Point Boulevard
PO Box 927
Elk Grove Village, IL 60007
(847) 228-5005
www.aap.org

The American Medical Association
515 North State Street
Chicago, IL 60610
(312) 464-5000
www.ama-assn.org

Asthma and Allergy Foundation of
America
1125 Fifteenth Street NW
Washington, DC 20005
(800) 7-ASTHMA
www.aafa.org

The Centers for Disease Control and
Prevention
1600 Clifton Road NE
Atlanta, GA 30333
(800) 311-3435
www.cdc.gov

National Cystic Fibrosis Foundation
60 East Forty-second Street
New York, NY 10165
(212) 986-8783
www.cff.org

National Institute of Allergy and
Infectious Disease
31 Center Drive MSC 2520
Bethesda, MD 20892
(301) 496-5717
www.niaid.nih.gov

National Institutes of Health
9000 Rockville Pike
Bethesda, MD 20892
(301) 496-4000
www.nih.gov

ACKNOWLEDGMENTS

The authors would like to take this opportunity to acknowledge the individuals who made this book possible. Many thanks to our agent, Judith Riven, who first saw the promise of this project and steered us through it. We are also deeply indebted to our editor at Holt, Deb Brody, whose invaluable expertise, vision, and advice helped shape this work into the final version you see before you today.

On a personal note, Shelagh would like to thank her daughter, Caitlin, both for her patience while her mother toiled for countless hours at the computer and for acting as an inadvertent inspiration for this book. Several years ago while visiting a new pediatrician, Shelagh was informed that Caitlin could not possibly have sinusitis—because sinusitis didn't exist! This provided an early insight into the many frustrating obstacles faced by sinusitis sufferers on a regular basis.

ABOUT THE AUTHORS

HARVEY PLASSE, M.D., is director of otolaryngology at the NYU Downtown Hospital, and associate professor of otolaryngology at the New York University School of Medicine.

SHELAGH RYAN MASLINE is an experienced health writer, the coauthor of multiple works of nonfiction, and a regular contributor to health journals.